DIABETIC
RETINOPATHY

DIABETIC

RETINOPATHY

Jean Daniel Arbour, M.D.

Pierre Labelle, M.D.

In collaboration with Frédérique David

Preface by Andrée Boucher, M.D.

AP Annika Parance Publishing

AP Annika Parance Publishing
1043 Marie-Anne Street East
Montreal, Quebec H2J 2B5
514-658-7217
apediteur.com

English translation: Debby Dubrofsky
Book and cover design: Francis Desrosiers in collaboration with Scalpel Design
Cover photograph: Istockphoto/Marianna Bettini

Photographs and illustrations courtesy of the Institut Nazareth & Louis-Braille
(pages 87, 89 and 92), Pierre Labelle, M.D. (pages 37, 41, 45, 63, 65 and 67)
and Novartis Pharma Canada Inc. (pages 31 and 47).

**Bibliothèque et Archives nationales du Québec and
Library and Archives Canada cataloguing in publication**

Arbour, Jean Daniel, 1964-
    Diabetic retinopathy
    (Understand the disease and its treatment)
    Translation of: La rétinopathie diabétique
    ISBN 978-2-923830-16-2

    1. Diabetic retinopathy - Popular works. 2. Diabetic retinopathy - Treat-
ment - Popular works. I. Labelle, Pierre, 1940-   . II. Title. III. Series:
Understand the disease and its treatment.

RE661.D5A7213 2013   617.7'35 C2013-940703-0

Legal deposit - Bibliothèque et Archives nationales du Québec, 2013
Legal deposit - Library and Archives Canada, 2013

© Annika Parance Publishing, 2013

This publication was made possible through an educational grant from Novartis
Pharma Canada Inc.

Printed in Canada

Over the years of our medical practice, we have met and treated a great many patients with diabetes and have become friends with some of them. For all of these people, the spectre of losing their sight, so precious to us all, looms large. The possibility of blindness is never far from their thoughts.

Fortunately, different treatments are now available, thanks to scientific breakthroughs. The prognosis for people with diabetic retinopathy is no longer what it was and we have reason to be optimistic about the future.

To all our diabetic patients, we affectionately dedicate this book.

Pierre Labelle and Jean Daniel Arbour

The authors would like to thank Annika Parance and Frédérique David for their tenacity, rigour and professionalism. Without them, this book would never have seen the light.

FROM THE SAME PUBLISHER
(apediteur.com)

In the same collection

Jean Daniel Arbour, M.D. and Pierre Labelle, M.D.
Diabetic Retinopathy (2013)
(French version: *La rétinopathie diabétique*)

Fadi Massoud, M.D. and Alain Robillard, M.D.
La maladie d'Alzheimer (2013)

Fred Saad, M.D. and Michael McCormack, M.D.
Prostate Cancer, 3rd edition (2012)
(French version: *Le cancer de la prostate*)

Jean Daniel Arbour, M.D., Francine Behar-Cohen, M.D.,
Pierre Labelle, M.D. and Florian Sennlaub, M.D.
AMD – Age-Related Macular Degeneration (2010)
(French version: *DMLA – La dégénérescence maculaire liée
à l'âge*)

CONTENTS

CHAPTER 2

FORMS AND SYMPTOMS OF DIABETIC RETINOPATHY 39

CHAPTER 3
CAUSES AND RISK FACTORS   49

CHAPTER 4
DIAGNOSIS   59

CHAPTER 5

PREVENTION AND TREATMENT 71

CHAPTER 6

LIVING WITH DIABETIC RETINOPATHY   **83**

CHAPTER 7

TREATMENTS OF THE FUTURE 97

LIST OF BOXES

THE AUTHORS

Jean Daniel Arbour, M.D.

Dr. Jean Daniel Arbour heads the ophthalmology department of the faculty of medicine at the University of Montreal, where he is also associate professor.

After receiving his M.D. from the University of Montreal, Dr. Arbour interned in general surgery, specialized in ophthalmology and then went to Harvard University in the United States for clinical and surgical retina training. At Harvard, Dr. Arbour also conducted research on macular degeneration and photodynamic and antiangiogenic therapy.

Dr. Arbour is currently vitreoretinal surgeon at Notre-Dame Hospital, which is part of the University of Montreal Hospital Centre (CHUM). He is also the founder of the hospital's ophthalmology research centre, where he has been the principal investigator in genetic studies of wet age-related macular degeneration (AMD) and numerous international studies of new treatments in macular degeneration and diabetic retinopathy.

The author of many articles published in medical journals, Dr. Arbour has also given more than 70 national and international scientific conferences on retinal disease.

Dr. Arbour was president of the Quebec association of ophthalmologists from 2005 to 2009 and treasurer of the Canadian

Ophthalmological Society from 2007 to 2010. He regularly serves as an expert for government bodies such as the INESSS (Quebec's national institute of excellence in health and social services) and the *Agence de santé de Montréal* (Montreal health agency).

Pierre Labelle, M.D.

Dr. Pierre Labelle is an ophthalmologist at Maisonneuve-Rosemont Hospital and full clinical professor in the department of ophthalmology of the faculty of medicine at the University of Montreal.

After receiving his M.D. and his diploma in ophthalmology, Dr. Labelle completed a research fellowship in retinal diseases and surgery at Washington University in St. Louis in the United States. He earned the first medal awarded by the Canadian Ophthalmological Society for his work on the prevention of sports-related eye injuries and was awarded the Securitas prize by the *Régie de la sécurité dans les sports du Québec*, Quebec's sports safety board, for his public awareness work. In 2010, he was granted a Lifetime Achievement Award by the Canadian Ophthalmological Society.

Dr. Labelle is president of the *Association des médecins ophtalmologistes du Québec*, Quebec's association of ophthalmologists, and heads the ophthalmology departments of Maisonneuve-Rosemont Hospital and the faculty of medicine of the University of Montreal. Under his direction, the Centre Michel-Mathieu was established at Maisonneuve-Rosemont Hospital in 1999, an internationally renowned institute of excellence in ophthalmology. Given his interest in clinical research, Dr. Labelle has collaborated on many research projects, including projects investigating diabetic retinopathy.

SPECIAL CONTRIBUTOR TO CHAPTER 6, LIVING WITH DR

Julie-Andrée Marinier

Optometrist and assistant professor at the school of optometry at the University of Montreal, Julie-Andrée Marinier also serves as low-vision optometrist at the Institut Nazareth & Louis-Braille (NLB) in Montreal.

She received her Doctor of Optometry degree and an M.Sc. in Vision Science from the University of Montreal. Her M.Sc. dissertation addresses the investigation of choroidal blood flow in age-related macular degeneration (AMD).

She has also contributed articles to medical journals and participated in numerous international conferences on low vision. She is especially interested in visual rehabilitation of people living with vision impairment.

PREFACE

With the changes in our lifestyle, the growth in obesity rates and
the sedentary lives we lead, diabetes is becoming more and more
common. Certain statistics suggest more than a third of the population of Canada has diabetes. One of the long-term complications
of diabetes is retinopathy, by far the most serious and most common eye disease associated with diabetes.

Poorly controlled blood sugar, diabetes of long date and subop-
mal blood pressure are risk factors for diabetic retinopathy (DR).
Diabetic retinopathy can take several forms. As it is asymptomatic
at the start, screening through regular eye examinations is crucial.
At a more advanced stage, diabetic retinopathy can lead to hemorrhaging, and treatment is required. It is at this point that there is a
risk of total or partial loss of vision.

This book by professors Jean Daniel Arbour, M.D., and Pierre
Labelle, M.D., offers clear explanations of this common disease. It
demystifies diabetic retinopathy. Above all, it gives hope to diabetics by suggesting ways of preventing this complication. The importance of good blood sugar, blood lipid and blood pressure control
in reducing the risk of developing these serious eye complications
cannot be overemphasized.

In addition to advice for preventing DR, this book also describes
tools to help manage the disease once it has arisen as well as

resources for those affected. It can help people with diabetes to better understand and manage their disease and to become a partner in taking charge of their health.

The patient as partner. It's a new paradigm very much in keeping with the way our society is evolving!

Andrée Boucher, M.D., FRCPC
Endocrinologist
University of Montreal Hospital Centre (CHUM)
Medical Director, Thyroid Cancer Team (CHUM)
Vice-Dean, Continuing Professional Development
Director, Health Sciences Teaching Centre (CPASS)
Faculty of Medicine, University of Montreal

25 FREQUENTLY ASKED QUESTIONS

(1) Is diabetic retinopathy (DR) a common disorder?

In Canada, 1.8 million people have type 1 or type 2 diabetes. DR is an eye complication of diabetes that affects 99 percent of people with type 2 diabetes and 60 percent of those with type 1 diabetes within 20 years of the onset of diabetes. DR is one of the leading causes of blindness in industrialized countries (Chapter 1).

(2) What are the symptoms of DR?

DR is a painless disease. Perceptible symptoms (the main one is vision loss) may not appear until late in the progression of the disease, when complications arise (Chapter 2).

(3) What causes DR?

Diabetic retinopathy, as its name indicates, is caused by diabetes. Hyperglycemia (high blood sugar) can cause the walls of the tiny blood vessels in the retina (retinal capillaries) to gradually become fragile, swell and leak fluid (plasma) and blood (Chapter 3).

(4) Does DR always progress at the same pace?

The progression of DR varies. It can, however, progress more quickly in case of poor blood sugar control, high blood pressure, pregnancy, puberty or cataract surgery (Chapters 2 and 3).

(5) What are the forms of DR?

There are two forms of DR: nonproliferative DR and proliferative DR. In nonproliferative DR, the blood vessels, which have become fragile due to an excess of blood sugar, start to leak fluid (plasma) and blood, and this can cause the retina to swell. In proliferative DR (an aggravation of nonproliferative DR) small abnormal blood vessels form, invading the retina. These blood vessels can break, causing hemorrhages (Chapter 2).

(6) What is macular edema?

Macular edema is a complication of nonproliferative as well as proliferative DR (and of other diseases, particularly vein occlusions). It is a swelling of the macula (the central area of the retina) caused by leakage of fluid and blood through the walls of dilated blood vessels. Macular edema is the most common cause of vision loss (Chapter 1).

(7) How do you know if you have DR?

As diabetic retinopathy is a disease that remains asymptomatic until a very advanced stage, the importance of regular eye examinations cannot be overemphasized, especially for people who are diabetic. An optometrist or ophthalmologist can detect DR by examining the back of the eye (ocular fundus examination), which will also indicate the type and severity of the disease (Chapters 4 and 5).

⑧ Does DR cause blindness?

Yes, but only in very rare cases. DR can cause blindness at a very advanced stage if necessary measures (screening, prevention and treatment) have not been taken in time (Chapter 5).

⑨ Can vision loss as a result of DR be prevented?

Yes. Vision loss can usually be prevented in people with diabetes by regular eye examinations throughout their lifetime. In addition, the better the diabetes control, the better the chances of preventing complications that could lead to vision impairment (Chapters 2 and 5).

⑩ When is an emergency visit required?

An emergency consultation with a vision specialist is required when a sudden major change in vision is noticed (Chapter 4).

⑪ Can DR be triggered by certain drugs?

To date, no drugs have been associated with the onset of DR. However, certain drugs promote dilation of blood vessels and can accelerate the progression of DR. Doctors know which drugs to avoid and, when necessary, will recommend more appropriate treatments (Chapter 3).

⑫ Can DR be prevented?

Diabetic retinopathy is a disease that can be prevented, mainly through the management of diabetes (Chapter 5).

⑬ Can DR be cured?

There is no treatment for the nonproliferative form of DR without macular edema, but its progression can sometimes be slowed by regular eye examinations and satisfactory management of diabetes and other aggravating disorders, such as high blood pressure. The proliferative form can be stopped. Available treatments can often lead to an improvement in vision (Chapter 5).

⑭ Can the progression of DR be slowed?

Yes. Existing therapies have proven effective in slowing the progression of symptoms of DR. Even better, certain treatments can actually improve vision (Chapter 5).

⑮ Can an operation be performed?

A vitrectomy, a surgical operation in which the vitreous humour is removed from the eye, can be performed in case of massive or chronic vitreal hemorrhage, retinal detachment and some cases of macular edema (Chapter 5).

⑯ If one eye is affected, will the other be automatically affected?

The signs and symptoms of DR can appear in one eye only, but usually both eyes are affected—though not necessarily equally (Chapter 2).

⑰ How often should a specialist be consulted?

Monitoring by an optometrist or an ophthalmologist is indispensable if you have DR. The treatment required and the frequency of visits will be determined by your vision specialist (Chapters 4 and 5).

⑱ Is DR painful?

No, DR is not painful. The eye examinations required and the treatments available are not painful either (Chapter 2).

⑲ Can you drive if you have DR?

Most people with DR keep their driver's licence. Corrected visual acuity must be at least 6/15 (20/50) to drive in Canada (Chapter 6).

⟨20⟩ Can you get around on your own if you have DR?

Yes. In the vast majority of cases, people with DR can get around on their own. Certain tools have been developed to make it easier for people with a vision impairment associated with advanced DR to get around (Chapter 6).

⟨21⟩ Are there vision aids that can help?

There are numerous vision aids (magnifiers, closed-circuit televisions, etc.) that facilitate daily activities for people with advanced DR (Chapter 6).

⟨22⟩ Is it possible to recover vision lost as a result of DR?

Yes. Vision often improves with treatment (laser photocoagulation, antiangiogenic drugs or vitrectomy). However, DR sometimes results in permanent vision loss (Chapter 5).

⟨23⟩ Should people with DR change their diet?

A very well-balanced diet and certain food guidelines are recommended for people with DR. Sugars and fats, which increase blood sugar levels, must be avoided (Chapters 3 and 5).

⟨24⟩ Should people with DR quit smoking?

It's always a good idea to quit smoking. Smokers are at greater risk of cardiovascular disease, high blood pressure in particular—a risk factor in DR (Chapters 3 and 5).

⟨25⟩ Will new treatments be able to cure DR?

New treatments available in the last few years have considerably improved the life of people with DR by slowing the progression of the disease and reducing symptoms. Research is ongoing, giving hope that future therapies will be even more effective in minimizing complications and perhaps, one day, preventing the disease—or at least delaying its onset (Chapter 7).

CHAPTER 1

UNDERSTANDING DIABETIC RETINOPATHY

Diabetic retinopathy (DR) is a disease of the retina caused by diabetes. It is also one of the leading causes of blindness among adults in industrialized countries. In Canada, 99 percent of people with type 1 diabetes and 60 percent of those with type 2 diabetes develop DR in the first 20 years after the onset of diabetes. An alarming increase in the number of people with diabetic retinopathy may be in the offing, as the worldwide diabetic population will double by 2030 (to more than 360 million people), according to the World Health Organization (WHO), if appropriate measures are not taken. Diabetic retinopathy is an insidious disease, as it can reach a very advanced stage without any loss of vision. Early detection has thus become a major issue in the fight against this disease, especially since there are very effective treatments available that can not only slow the progression of the disease but can even restore lost vision.

WHAT IS DIABETIC RETINOPATHY?

Diabetic retinopathy, as its name indicates, is associated with diabetes (*see Chapter 3, Causes and risk factors*). It occurs when hyperglycemia (high blood sugar) over time causes the walls of the tiny blood vessels in the retina (retinal capillaries) to gradually become fragile. Generally both eyes are affected, but not necessarily equally. DR always begins in the nonproliferative form and may progress to the proliferative form.

In nonproliferative (or background) diabetic retinopathy, the blood vessels of the retina dilate and leak blood and fluid, causing the retina to "swell."

In the proliferative form of DR, small abnormal blood vessels invade the retina to compensate for the reduced blood circulation. These abnormal blood vessels are fragile, however, and tend to break easily, causing hemorrhaging.

DR is a disease that can be controlled, mainly through the management of diabetes. It can be stabilized and its progression stopped. Left untreated, however, diabetic retinopathy often leads to permanent vision loss and ultimately blindness. It is thus crucial that diabetic retinopathy be diagnosed as early as possible, so it can be properly followed and treated in a timely fashion.

As diabetic retinopathy is painless and symptoms may not appear until late in the course of the disease, the only way of detecting diabetic retinopathy early is regular eye examinations.

HOW THE EYE AND THE RETINA WORK

A brief explanation of how the eye works will help in understanding how diabetic retinopathy affects vision.

The eye is a spherical organ about 2.5 centimetres (one inch) in diameter consisting of several covering layers plus internal structures (*Figure* ❶). Only part of the eye is visible; the rest is hidden inside the skull. The eye is often said to work like a 35-millimetre camera (before the advent of digital cameras): to get a clear, crisp

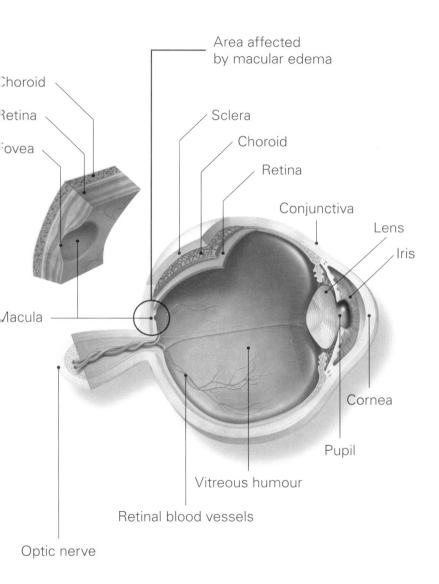

Area affected
by macular edema

Choroid

Retina

Fovea

Sclera

Choroid

Retina

Conjunctiva

Lens

Iris

Macula

Cornea

Pupil

Vitreous humour

Retinal blood vessels

Optic nerve

Cross section of the eye

image, we adjust the focus and then the diaphragm opens and closes to let in the right amount of light. The same principle applies to the eye. The image is focused by the cornea and the lens, and the iris serves as the diaphragm. The image thus formed is projected onto the retina, which lines the back of the eye like film in a traditional roll-film camera.

The sclera and the conjunctiva

The sclera (the white of the eye) is the tough outer wall that surrounds and protects the eye. The optic nerve is attached to the sclera at the back of the eye. The visible part of the sclera is covered by a thin, transparent membrane, the conjunctiva, which folds forward to become the lining of the inside of the eyelid.

The cornea

The cornea is the transparent membrane at the front of the eye covering the eye like the glass that covers the face of a watch. About a half millimetre thick, the cornea forms a clear dome over the iris, from which it is separated by aqueous fluid. The cornea controls the entry of light, protecting the inside of the eye by partially blocking ultraviolet rays. In advanced diabetes, corneal sensitivity is reduced (diminished perception of tactile sensations or pain). Corneal transparency is also reduced, and this can lead to vision loss (blurred vision).

The iris and the pupil

The iris is the visible coloured part of the eye. At its centre is an opening, the pupil, which allows light to enter the eye and reach the retina. Like the aperture in a camera, the iris controls the amount of light going into the eye depending on the ambient lighting. The pupil contracts and dilates to regulate the amount of light that reaches the retina. Advanced diabetic retinopathy can cause growth of new abnormal blood vessels on the iris, known as rubeosis. Rubeosis can lead to glaucoma, an eye disease characterized by elevated interocular pressure that can mean gradual loss of vision.

The lens

The lens is located behind the iris. The role of the lens is to focus images projected onto the back of the eye. To do this, the lens changes shape depending on the distance between the eye and the object viewed. With age, the lens loses its flexibility and cannot change shape as easily. This results in presbyopia, a condition in which the eye loses its ability to focus on near objects.

In people with diabetes, a particular type of cataract (clouding of the lens) often occurs that progresses rapidly, causing increased sensitivity to bright light and major glare symptoms. The significant fluctuations in blood sugar level (glycemia) over the course of a day in people whose diabetes is poorly controlled can affect the lens, sometimes causing rapid though temporary changes in vision—such as myopia, which affects distance vision.

The vitreous humour

Between the lens and the retina, the eye is filled with a transparent gelatinous substance (like the white of an egg) called the vitreous humour, the vitreous body or the vitreous. The vitreous occupies about 80 percent of the volume of the eyeball. It is transparent, allowing light to travel to the retina, and it also transports nutrients important for the health of the eye.

Hemorrhaging in the vitreous (intravitreal hemorrhage) is common in people with diabetic retinopathy and the resulting vision loss depends on the scope of the hemorrhaging. For a clear image, the vitreous must be free of hemorrhages.

The retina

The retina is a thin film of nerve tissue lining 75 percent of the inner surface of the eyeball. Here is where the photoreceptors are located, the cells that convert light to nerve impulses delivered to the brain by the optic nerve. The leaking blood vessels and hemorrhages in the retina that are characteristic of diabetic retinopathy can cause a decrease in visual acuity.

The macula

The macula is a very small area (about two millimetres in diameter) at the centre of the retina. The macula transmits 90 percent of the visual information processed by the brain. Composed of closely packed photoreceptor cells, the macula is responsible for fine detail vision (such as reading and recognizing faces) as well as colour detection. The retina as a whole allows us to see the book on the table, for example, but the macula makes it possible for us to read the words in the book. The macula is also called the "yellow spot" because of its yellow colour, due to a high concentration of lutein, an antioxidant of the carotenoid family. In people with diabetic retinopathy, the macula may swell, causing blurred vision (see box, *What is macular edema?*).

The fovea

The fovea is a small dimple a half millimetre in diameter at the centre of the macula, the region of greatest visual acuity (responsible for high-resolution vision). The fovea is the centre of the eye's sharpest vision. It is also largely responsible for colour vision, thanks to its densely packed cones (photoreceptors). The closer a hemorrhage or edema (swelling) is to the fovea, the more devastating the central vision loss.

The optic nerve

Located at the back of the eye, the optic nerve transmits visual information to the brain. At birth, the optic nerve is composed of roughly one million nerve fibres, called axons, that stretch from the ganglion cells of the retina out the eyeball into the brain. In people with diabetic retinopathy, new abnormal blood vessels (neovessels) may appear on the optic nerve.

Oculomotor nerves

There are twelve pairs of cranial nerves, most of which originate in the brainstem, the part of the brain just above the spinal cord. These nerves have sensory and/or motor functions, which means they play a role in vision and in eye movement. Three of the twelve cranial nerves control the six muscles that allow the eye to move in all directions. These nerves can be affected by blood circulation disorders caused by diabetes, leading to misalignment of the two eyes and causing double vision (diplopia). Fortunately, this is generally temporary and disappears on its own within months or weeks (*see Chapter 2*). Other disorders, however, some of them very serious, can also cause sudden double vision. As a result, it is important to see a doctor quickly if you start to see double to determine the cause.

Blood circulation in the eye

The eye is supplied with blood by the ophthalmic artery, which passes through the optic nerve and then divides into several branches that supply different parts of the eye—including the posterior ciliary arteries, which supply the choroid, and the central

WHAT IS MACULAR EDEMA?

Macular edema is a complication of DR that can arise in the nonproliferative or the proliferative form of DR. It may also be associated with other eye diseases—particularly vein occlusions, which result from sudden blockage of venous circulation in the retina. Macular edema is the most common cause of vision loss in diabetic retinopathy. It is a swelling of the macula (the central area of the retina) caused by fluid or blood leaking through the walls of dilated blood vessels. These leaks and/or hemorrhages cause a significant loss of visual acuity, as the macula is the part of the retina responsible for fine detail vision—needed for reading, driving and watching television, for example. Fortunately, the vision loss caused by macular edema is often reversible. In fact, new treatments are now available (*see Chapter 5*) that can improve the vision of people with diabetic macular edema.

artery of the retina. The retina thus receives its nutrition from two discrete circulatory systems:

- The choroidal blood vessels, which carry blood (and hence oxygen) to the outer layers of the retina (pigment epithelium, photoreceptors)
- The retinal blood vessels, which supply the inner layers of the retina with blood and oxygen

The central artery of the retina branches out into a network of blood vessels ending in the retinal capillaries (tiny blood vessels).

In DR, it is the retinal blood vessels that are affected. The choroidal circulatory system can also be affected in people with diabetes, a disorder called diabetic choroidopathy.

HOW WE SEE

Light passes first through the cornea, the aqueous humour, the lens and the vitreous humour before falling on the retina. It is there, not in the brain, that processing of the image by the nervous system begins. In fact, many anatomists consider the retina an extension of the brain. As thin as a sheet of paper, the retina (*Figure* ❷) is nonetheless more complex and more sensitive than photographic film. It has ten distinct layers, each with a specific function and each liable to be affected by DR. Light must cross several of these layers to reach the 125 million photoreceptors (light-sensitive cells) that absorb the light and convert it to nerve impulses, which are relayed to the brain via the optic nerve.

The role of the photoreceptors

The retina contains two types of photoreceptors (rods and cones), and each plays a different role in the perception of images.

There are approximately 120 million rods in each eye, and they are sensitive to dim light, allowing us to see at night. During the day, or in bright light, the rods stop responding. Rods cannot resolve

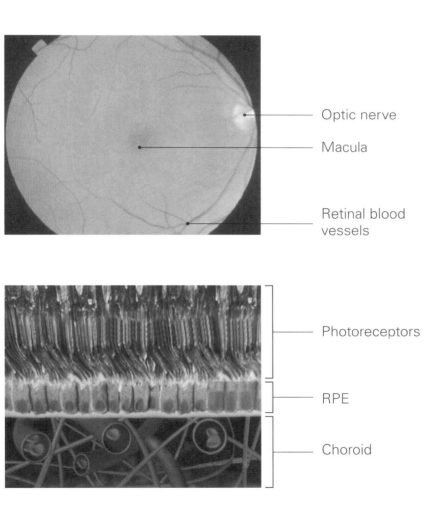

Optic nerve

Macula

Retinal blood vessels

Photoreceptors

RPE

Choroid

❷ Normal retina

fine detail or distinguish colours, but they are responsible for peripheral vision.

There are fewer cones (five million), but their capacity to distinguish detail is one hundred times greater than that of the rods. Very numerous in the macula, cones are responsible for colour vision and are used mainly in bright light (during the day or with artificial lighting). Cones are tuned to different portions of the colour spectrum: some perceive blue, others red and still others green. The cones are responsible for fine detail vision.

Photoreceptors are extremely fragile. To transmit a clear and accurate image, they must not be disturbed by edema, hemorrhages or retinal detachment, all of which can occur in diabetic retinopathy.

The role of the retinal pigment epithelium (RPE)

The retinal pigment epithelium (RPE) is a single layer of cells under the retina. One of the roles of the RPE is to remove waste from the retina that is produced by the photoreceptors when converting light to nerve impulses. Diabetic retinopathy can affect the RPE.

The role of the choroid

Located under the retina, the choroid supplies the photoreceptors with the oxygen and nourishment they require to function properly. Though relatively small (a single layer of organic tissue), the choroid contains very large blood vessels and blood flow through these vessels is greater than anywhere else in the body—demonstrating the extent to which the photoreceptors need nourishment to function properly. When diabetes affects the blood vessels of the choroid, the disorder is called diabetic choroidopathy.

CHAPTER 2
FORMS
AND SYMPTOMS
OF DIABETIC
RETINOPATHY

There are two forms of diabetic retinopathy (DR). Nonproliferative or background retinopathy develops first. This is the early stage of diabetic retinopathy, which can progress to the proliferative or advanced form of the disease. DR is a deceptive disease, as it does not cause any symptoms at first, only signs that can be detected solely in an eye examination by a health professional. Vision disorders generally only appear when complications of the disease arise, such as macular edema, hemorrhaging, neovascular glaucoma or retinal detachment—at which point the visual impairment can be substantial and lead to blindness. It is, however, possible to avoid these complications by early detection of DR and satisfactory management of general health (diabetes, blood pressure, smoking cessation, etc.).

NONPROLIFERATIVE DR

In the nonproliferative or background form of DR, too much sugar in the blood as a result of diabetes causes the normally impermeable walls of the retinal blood vessels to dilate and become permeable. Elevated blood sugar alters the response of the cells that line the inside of the blood vessels, causing their deterioration. This results in the formation of microaneurysms, tiny areas of swelling of the blood vessels, and this can lead to microhemorrhaging, that is, leaking of fluid (plasma) and blood into the retina. The number of leaks gradually increases over time, leading to edema (swelling) of the retina—and a decrease in visual acuity if the edema affects the macula (the central part of the retina).

About 25 percent of people who have had type 1 diabetes for five to ten years or type 2 diabetes for ten years will develop nonproliferative DR.

Signs and symptoms

The earliest signs of the nonproliferative form of DR are small spots on the retina which can be detected only in an examination of the back of the eye (fundoscopy) performed by a health professional (optometrist, family doctor, ophthalmologist, endocrinologist or other medical specialist) (*see Chapter 4*). These spots may be microaneurysms, or the fluid or blood leaks microaneurysms cause, or they may be white deposits of blood lipids (exudates)— that is, fatty matter that is normally not found outside the blood stream (*Figure* ❶). These lesions may appear in one or both eyes, and they can also disappear spontaneously, without treatment when blood sugar balance is achieved.

The nonproliferative form of DR is generally asymptomatic. Early retina damage often does not affect vision unless the macula is affected (see box, *The symptoms of macular edema*). Nonproliferative

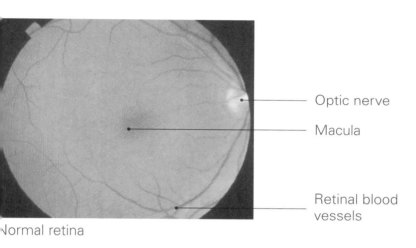

Optic nerve

Macula

Retinal blood vessels

Normal retina

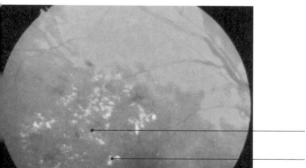

Microaneurysms

Lipids

Nonproliferative diabetic retinopathy (DR)

DR is not painful and usually does not cause any loss of vision—or at least generally not any perceptible loss. To prevent macular edema or progression to the proliferative form of DR, people with diabetes must have their eyes examined regularly. Ophthalmological monitoring and satisfactory management of diabetes can reduce the probability of one day developing the proliferative form of the disease. However, it is important to understand that there are no hard and fast rules for the progression of the disease. Even when diabetes is well controlled, DR can progress from the nonproliferative to the proliferative form at any time and there is no way to prevent this from happening. Nonetheless, the risk is lower when doctors' recommendations are followed.

PROLIFERATIVE DR

Proliferative DR is the more advanced form of the disease. Not only do the blood vessels swell and leak fluid or blood, as in the nonproliferative form of the disease, but new abnormal blood vessels grow on the surface of the retina, a process termed neovascularization. These new abnormal vessels, or neovessels, appear because blood flow is inadequate in the damaged blood vessels of the retina, causing the retina to become oxygen deficient (ischemic). In other words, normal blood circulation is required to ensure a constant supply of oxygen and essential nutrients to all parts of the eye, including the retina. When low blood sugar affects blood circulation to the eye, new abnormal blood vessels develop to compensate for the insufficient supply of blood and the accompanying oxygen deficiency.

The new abnormal blood vessels multiply on the surface of the retina, sometimes invading the surface of the optic nerve as well and eventually the vitreous humour and even the iris. These vessels are fragile and cause hemorrhages when they break.

As many as 25 percent of patients who have had type 1 diabetes for 15 years and 10 percent of patients with type 2 diabetes for 15 years will develop proliferative DR. Prevalence is higher among patients with type 1 diabetes.

The disease may progress more quickly in case of poor blood sugar control, high blood pressure, pregnancy, puberty or cataract surgery (*see Chapter 3*).

Signs and symptoms

In the proliferative form of DR, as in the nonproliferative form, symptoms only appear when complications arise. Without complications, the only signs of proliferative DR are those that an eye care health professional might detect on examining the back of the eye. These are the same signs as those that appear with nonproliferative DR, but there will also be abnormal blood vessels growing along the surface of the retina (*Figure ❷*). These abnormal blood vessels require treatment.

When vision loss is perceived, it is generally related to one of the four possible complications of proliferative DR: macular edema (see box, *The symptoms of macular edema*), vitreous hemorrhage or, more rarely, neovascular glaucoma or retinal detachment. The symptoms may appear in one eye only, as the complications do not necessarily affect both eyes. In addition, both eyes are rarely affected in the same way, which means the vision loss may not be the same in both eyes.

Vitreous hemorrhage

Vitreous hemorrhage occurs when an abnormal blood vessel (neovessel) breaks, causing blood to flow inside the eye into one of the spaces formed within and around the vitreous body. The hemorrhage may be very small or massive, and the symptoms will depend on the size of the hemorrhage. A mild hemorrhage will cause "floaters" to appear in the field of vision. These floaters are often described as lines or spider webs and the amount depends on the quantity of bleeding in the vitreous. A severe hemorrhage can cause a sudden major but painless loss of vision in the eye (perception of light only).

Fortunately, this sudden blindness is reversible. With time the hemorrhage may resorb spontaneously. If it doesn't, surgery (vitrectomy) can be considered. Vision then improves after a period of recovery which varies from case to case (*see Chapter 5*).

Retinal detachment

Proliferation of new abnormal vessels on the retina, especially when accompanied by vitreal hemorrhaging, can provoke a repair process that leads to formation of fibrous membranes between the vitreous humour and the retina. These membranes produce mechanical traction on the retina and can pull on it till it detaches. Fortunately, the disease rarely progresses to this stage among people with diabetes.

Retinal detachment can cause major vision loss, including permanent blindness, though this is very rare. This complication is not painful, presenting as a sudden or gradual vision loss proportional to the detachment—which can be peripheral, central or total. Rapid treatment is required.

Neovascular glaucoma

Neovascular glaucoma arises when abnormal blood vessels proliferate in the angle between the iris and the cornea (the iridocorneal angle) and on the surface of the iris (rubeosis). These abnormal blood vessels may lead to obstruction of the angle, preventing drainage of the aqueous humour and causing a sudden increase in intraocular pressure, sometimes accompanied by acute eye pain and headache. Neovascular glaucoma can cause a sudden or gradual vision loss. This serious, though fortunately rare, complication requires emergency consultation of an ophthalmologist.

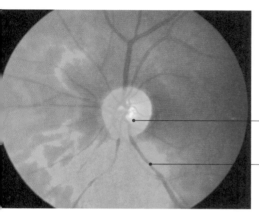

Optic nerve

Retinal blood vessels

Normal retina

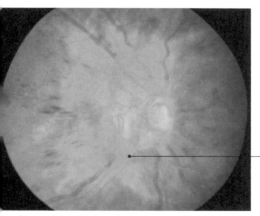

Neovascularization

Proliferative diabetic retinopathy (DR)

THE SYMPTOMS OF MACULAR EDEMA

As macular edema is a disorder of the macula, it affects fine detail vision (see box, *What is macular edema? in Chapter 1*). This complication, which may occur in both forms of DR, can thus cause significant central vision loss (peripheral vision is spared) in one or both eyes, making it impossible to read, recognize faces or drive. Vision loss as a result of macular edema is painless and generally gradual, though the onset may be sudden in rare cases. The vision loss may not be the same in both eyes if both are affected. Macular edema generally causes blurred vision, as if the eye can no longer focus on the image. Some people also experience metamorphopsia, that is, object distortion in which straight lines become wavy (*Figure ❸*). Fortunately, treatments are available that generally result in recovery of vision, but the treatments often have to be repeated at variable intervals (*see Chapter 5*).

There are no symptoms that can warn people with DR that macular edema is to be anticipated. By the time central vision is lost, macular edema has already developed. It is nonetheless possible to prevent macular edema by keeping blood sugar down to a reasonable level and controlling modifiable risk factors for diabetes. Though macular edema can develop even when diabetes is properly managed, it is generally possible to prevent the progression of DR to complications such as macular edema by consistent management of blood sugar, weight, blood pressure, smoking and so forth. The better the diabetes control, the better the chances of preventing this complication.

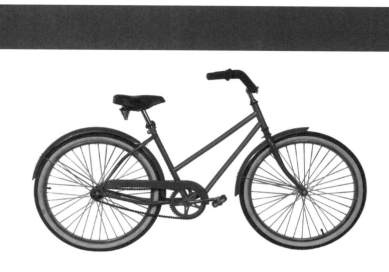

Normal vision

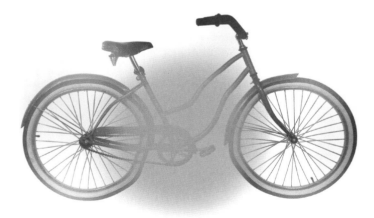

Vision with macular edema

ONE PERSON'S STORY

Name: Clara | **Age:** 71 years old

Occupation: Teacher, retired

Clara retired from teaching at the age of 60. She leads an active life today, despite some health issues that are now well under control. In the first year of her retirement, when she went to the hospital for pain that proved to be angina pectoris, a blood test showed she had type 2 diabetes. An ophthalmologist subsequently diagnosed proliferative diabetic retinopathy (DR) in both eyes. The disease had progressed over the years without Clara being aware of it because the symptoms were virtually imperceptible and completely painless.

Before her retirement, Clara had been completely absorbed in her work and she had neglected her health. She was overweight and not physically active. A year after retiring, she noticed a vision loss, but she attributed it to aging. She was having difficulty seeing clearly not only at a distance but also up close. In addition, spots in her central vision were blurry and less sharp. She was having more and more trouble reading and writing. Clara's ophthalmologist confirmed that her diabetes dated back a number of years and had affected both eyes. In fact, she had macular edema, a complication of DR. Fortunately, after several monthly injections of antiangiogenics, optical coherence tomography (OCT) showed the macular edema had disappeared, and Clara's vision improved substantially. Since then, Clara has been seeing her ophthalmologist regularly, so he can monitor the progression of her DR.

Clara has understood that diabetes is a real threat to her health and her eyesight, especially if she does not change her lifestyle habits. She has begun an exercise program with some friends and is taking the advice of a nutritionist at the CLSC to prevent her DR from progressing to a more advanced stage with new complications. She is happy she has decided to take her diabetes seriously and to maintain her eyesight.

CHAPTER 3
CAUSES AND
RISK FACTORS

Diabetic retinopathy (DR) is a direct complication of diabetes. In other words, the risk factors for diabetes are also those associated with the onset of DR. Other factors can accelerate the progression of the disease, particularly the duration of diabetes, poor blood sugar control and high blood pressure. A number of the risk factors for DR are modifiable, such as obesity and physical inactivity, which means it is possible to reduce the incidence and slow the progression of the disease by changing certain behaviours and lifestyle habits. Assiduous monitoring of diabetes and regular follow-up are thus crucial in managing the risk factors of DR.

CAUSE OF DR

DR is caused by type 2 and type 1 diabetes.

Type 1 diabetes is an autoimmune disease (due to abnormal action of the immune system) involving complete destruction of the cells of the pancreas responsible for producing insulin. Insulin is a hormone that allows glucose (from food) to be absorbed and used as "fuel" (that is, as a source of energy) by the cells of the body. People with type 1 diabetes do not produce insulin and must inject insulin several times a day, as insulin cannot be taken in the form of an oral medication (by mouth).

Type 2 diabetes is much more common (90 percent of all cases of diabetes) and it is often very insidious. A genetic predisposition, excess weight and lack of physical activity are contributing factors. In type 2 diabetes, the pancreas does not produce enough insulin and the cells of the body become resistant to the hormone's action.

In both types of diabetes, the insulin deficiency and/or resistance leads to abnormally high blood glucose (sugar) levels (or hyperglycemia). If insufficient insulin is produced, it cannot do its job properly, and glucose cannot be used to fuel the cells of the body. Instead, glucose accumulates in the blood, causing hyperglycemia—which can lead to complications that affect the eyes. DR is one of these complications.

WHAT IS A RISK FACTOR?

A risk factor does not, in and of itself, cause a disease. Its presence increases the probability that the disease will develop, especially when other risk factors are present as well. However, the presence of risk factors is no guarantee that the disease will actually develop. In other words, several risk factors may be present, yet the disease may never develop. On the other hand, the disease may develop even when no risk factors are present.

RISK FACTORS

A number of factors increase the risk of onset and progression of DR. Though some of these are nonmodifiable, such as genetics and ethnic origin, others can be controlled—elevated blood sugar, for example, and high blood pressure. It is thus important to pay attention to these modifiable risk factors so as not to aggravate existing diabetic retinopathy.

Duration of diabetes

Duration of diabetes is the strongest predictor of the development of DR and its severity. In Canada, 99 percent of people with type 1 diabetes and 60 percent with type 2 diabetes develop diabetic retinopathy in the first 20 years after the onset of diabetes.

Poor glycemic control

Development of DR is associated with elevated blood sugar (hyperglycemia), which causes the blood vessels of the retina to deteriorate (*see Chapter 2*). Poor blood sugar control increases the incidence of DR and the progression of disease symptoms. A major study (DCCT, published in 1993) compared the risk of developing DR in a group of patients who kept blood glucose levels virtually normal with the risk in a group whose average blood sugar levels were higher. This study clearly demonstrated that good blood sugar control reduces the risk of developing DR by up to 85 percent and the risk of its progression by up to 66 percent.

High blood pressure

Hypertension, or high blood pressure, is a major risk factor for DR. Hypertension causes the small arteries of the retina to harden, interfering with blood circulation in this part of the eye. Poorly controlled hypertension significantly increases the risk of aggravation of DR.

Heredity

The importance of heredity as a risk factor in diabetes depends on the type of diabetes concerned, type 1 or type 2. When one parent has type 2 diabetes, the risk of its transmission to offspring is 10 to 30 percent (30 to 60 percent if both parents have type 2 diabetes). However, when one parent has type 1 diabetes, the risk of transmission to offspring is only 5 percent (30 percent if both parents have type 1 diabetes).

To date, no specific gene has been identified as responsible for type 1 or type 2 diabetes. The disease seems to be multigenic, that, is several genes seem to be involved.

Hereditary factors that play a role in the development of diabetes are risk factors for DR.

High cholesterol (hypercholesterolemia)

Cholesterol refers to fatty substances (lipids) found in the blood. An elevated cholesterol level (hypercholesterolemia) is associated with fatty deposits on the walls of all blood vessels in the body, including those of the retina. These deposits interfere with blood circulation. Hypercholesterolemia is a risk factor in the development of complications such as DR in diabetics. Controlling blood cholesterol level thus helps to reduce the risk.

Ethnic origin

The risk of DR is higher in people of Aboriginal, Latin American, Asian, South Asian and African origin, in whom the incidence of diabetes is higher than among people of other ethnic origins, mainly for hereditary reasons. DR is particularly problematic among Canada's Aboriginal populations, where the prevalence of diabetes is at least three times as high as in the general population. About 30 to 40 percent of diabetic Aboriginals in Canada have DR, and 2.5 percent have proliferative DR.

Excess weight

Studies show a link between elevated body mass index (BMI) and progression of DR. We know that type 2 diabetes is more common in people who are overweight. This is because excess weight leads to insulin resistance. The higher the amount of fat in a person's body, the greater the need for insulin. We also know that lack of physical activity causes elevated blood sugar, which promotes hyperglycemia.

According to the World Health Organization (WHO), a person is overweight when his or her BMI is 25 or over and obese when it is 30 or over. BMI is the ratio of a person's weight to his or her height, and it provides an estimation of the risk of developing diseases associated with being overweight such as diabetes. At a healthy weight, BMI is between 18.5 and 24.9.

Sedentary lifestyle

Physical inactivity increases the risk of developing diabetes and thus DR, as it increases the risk of becoming overweight or obese—especially when combined with an unhealthy diet. According to the National Population Health Survey (NPHS), people who

WATCH OUT FOR PROTEINURIA!

Kidney health problems are closely related to eye health problems and vice versa. This means that eye complications can coincide with kidney impairments such as proteinuria. A simple analysis of a urine sample will detect proteinuria, or presence of proteins in the urine, which normally contains very little protein. Proteinuria can be a sign of more serious health problems. Thus, an ophthalmologist who detects DR will recommend follow-up for possible kidney problems. Likewise, when proteinuria is diagnosed in an annual checkup, an examination of the back of the eye is recommended. In fact, 60 to 90 percent of people with type 1 diabetes who are found to have proteinuria also have DR. And when proteinuria develops in someone who already has DR, it can be a sign of progression to proliferative DR.

expend no more than 1.5 kcal/kg/day (the equivalent of less than 15 minutes walking) are considered physically inactive.

Certain medications

Some medications promote dilation of blood vessels and can increase the symptoms and the progression of DR. These medications can provoke macular edema (*see Chapter 1*) in people with DR. Among the medications of concern are cortisone (which not only causes blood vessels to dilate but also increases blood sugar level) and certain pharmaceutical preparations used in the treatment of glaucoma. Closer blood sugar monitoring is required when these medications are taken. Doctors prescribe appropriate medication for each patient on a case-by-case basis.

Pregnancy

Pregnancy can cause blood sugar to increase, as the placenta produces hormones that check the action of insulin. This can lead to hyperglycemia and then pregnancy diabetes (gestational diabetes). This type of diabetes occurs in 2 to 4 percent of pregnancies and disappears after childbirth in 90 percent of those affected. It is not associated with DR.

However, in diabetic women, pregnancy can provoke DR (which often resolves after the pregnancy) or accelerate the progression of existing DR. It is important to emphasize that pregnancy-related DR only develops in women who were diabetic before becoming pregnant. In most cases, however, the condition of the retina improves immediately after childbirth and visual acuity is totally or partially recovered.

Diabetic women must consult their ophthalmologists in the first weeks of pregnancy. If DR is present at the start of the pregnancy, then closer ophthalmological monitoring is required. Some medications used to treat DR (antiangiogenics) cannot be used during pregnancy. Laser treatments, however, are completely safe (*see Chapter 5*).

Puberty

Although DR tends not to develop in diabetic children, it is common during puberty and can progress rapidly at that time. Growth hormones, which are very active during puberty, can alter the effect of insulin and increase blood sugar levels. In addition, this is a critical period, as compliance with diabetes follow-up and treatment can be problematic at this age, when risk-taking behaviour is the norm.

Increased monitoring of the eyes of young diabetics is required at puberty and during adolescence.

Cataract surgery

It has been clearly demonstrated that cataract surgery can cause DR to progress, as this surgery, like any operation, causes inflammation and can aggravate the existing inflammation in people with DR. In addition, macular edema can develop when the inflammation is located in the macula, a fragile part of the retina, and vision loss can result. In fact, even people who are not diabetic can develop macular edema as a result of cataract surgery.

Smoking

Studies suggest that smoking increases the risk of DR in people with type 1 diabetes. We also know that smoking increases the risk of cardiovascular disease, particularly hypertension, which is a risk factor in DR. Furthermore, nicotine, one of the components of tobacco, is an angiogenic, that is, it stimulates development of new abnormal blood vessels, which can aggravate DR. Although the role of smoking in the progression of DR remains controversial, it is a modifiable risk factor that it would be wise not to ignore.

Socioeconomic factors

According to the Public Health Agency of Canada, socioeconomic factors (education and income) have a major impact on the adoption of healthy behaviours. Several studies demonstrate that people with low incomes and little education are at a higher risk of smoking, being physically inactive, being overweight and denying the presence of the disease (see box, *Diabetes denial*). We know, however, that medical follow-up, glycemic control and a healthy lifestyle are essential in DR to prevent vision deterioration.

DIABETES DENIAL

Denial (categorical refusal to acknowledge the disease) is not rare among diabetics. It can be outright or unconscious, reflected in a refusal to follow doctors' instructions, accept medical care or change harmful habits (unhealthy diet). Denial is especially disturbing as it can delay the diagnosis of DR—to be discovered only when it has reached the advanced stage (proliferative DR). When denial is coupled with continuation of unhealthy lifestyle habits, diabetes can be aggravated and DR may develop earlier than if those lifestyle habits had been modified. Denial can take the form of an unbalanced diet, failure to take medication and lack of medical follow-up. It can also mean failure to regularly monitor one's eyes—with an eye examination every year or every two years, as recommended for people with diabetes. Some people deny the disease because they feel it is restrictive. Others feel invincible. Still others don't understand the importance of following their doctors' recommendations, especially when they don't have any symptoms.

Denial is especially frequent among adolescents. They deny their diabetes out of fear of being excluded, of appearing different, but also because the monitoring and restrictions imposed by the disease interfere with their freedom. In addition, adolescence is a time of recklessness, of risk-taking, when we don't really understand that our behaviour can have serious consequences.

Alcohol

Though there is little proof of any association between alcohol and DR, a review of 32 studies conducted between 1966 and 2003 showed that excessive alcohol consumption (more than three glasses a day) can be associated with an increase of up to 43 percent in the incidence of diabetes. Drinking in moderation is thus recommended.

ONE PERSON'S STORY

Name: Philip	**Age:** 51 years old

Occupation: IT professional

Phillip is a freelance IT consultant. He works long hours and is a big fan of fast food. Though he is not obese, he is very overweight and does little physical exercise. His family doctor told him five years ago that his blood pressure was too high and that he was at risk for type 2 diabetes, like his father and his brother. He admits that he failed to follow his doctor's advice: lose weight by eating better and start a physical exercise program; otherwise he must take medication.

Last year, Philip suddenly started to get worried when he noticed his vision deteriorating. He was afraid he would no longer be able to read documents on his computer screen or drive a car. He consulted an optometrist—who referred him to an ophthalmologist when he observed bleeding in Philip's retina on examining the back of his eye. The ophthalmologist diagnosed proliferative diabetic retinopathy (DR) with macular edema and signs of high blood pressure in the eyes. The disease was stabilized with antiangiogenic therapy and laser photocoagulation and Philip's vision improved. He consulted his family doctor again, who prescribed therapy for his diabetes and his high blood pressure and put him in contact with the team at a diabetes clinic.

Today, Philip eats a balanced diet, avoids sugar and exercises regularly. Since he has lost weight, he feels much better and his diabetes is easier to control. His vision is excellent and he sees his ophthalmologist for regular checkups. Philip understands now that he almost lost much of his vision and that he could have become blind, as his father did near the end of his life.

CHAPTER 4

DIAGNOSIS

Many health practitioners play a role in evaluating and monitoring eye and vision problems. Both optometrists and ophthalmologists are qualified to detect diabetic retinopathy (DR).

Diagnosis of DR in people with diabetes is based on detecting signs associated with DR (microaneurysms, hemorrhages, macular edema, neovascularization, etc.). The purpose of screening for DR is to prevent the visual impairment it can cause by early identification and suitable intervention. Early diagnosis is especially important because DR is a disease without any symptoms in the early stages. Many people are not aware that they have DR. An examination of the back of the eye (fundus examination) is required for a diagnosis to be made. After that, the ophthalmologist uses a variety of tests, performed in a private clinic or hospital, to determine the form of DR (proliferative or nonproliferative) and appropriate therapy.

EARLY DETECTION

Early detection of DR is crucial, so treatment can begin as soon as possible. There are recognized and effective treatments that can prevent the progression of DR and reduce the risk of blindness. However, the treatments work better when the diagnosis is made early and they are administered in a timely fashion.

Everyone diagnosed with diabetes must be followed regularly. Though it is essential to consult an ophthalmologist if you are diagnosed with type 1 diabetes, it is less urgent than if you are diagnosed with type 2 diabetes. RD does not generally develop in type 1 diabetes until years after the onset of the disease. With type 2 diabetes, which is generally well established before becoming apparent, an eye care professional must be consulted immediately on diagnosis, as RD may already be present. People with diabetes must consult an ophthalmologist every year, or every two years, as recommended.

We cannot insist too much on the importance of eye examinations, even when vision seems normal. Changes associated with RD can be detected during a routine eye examination even before symptoms appear. There are even people who learn they have diabetes when they receive a diagnosis of DR from their ophthalmologist.

COMPREHENSIVE EYE EXAMINATION

As part of the eye examination, a technician or vision specialist (optometrist or ophthalmologist) takes note of past health problems and performs certain tests. There are several steps before the back of the eye is examined (fundus examination).

General health and eye health questionnaire

In addition to recent symptoms and the fact that the patient is diabetic, it is important to know the patient's state of health (high blood pressure, heart disease, allergies, etc.), family history and any treatment or medication he or she is taking.

Visual acuity test

Vision is measured using a visual acuity chart called the Snellen chart or scale. The chart consists of rows of letters or drawings that decrease in size line by line. Vision specialists are referring to this chart when they speak of a gain or loss of a "line of visual acuity."

Visual acuity tests measure the sharpness of central vision, needed for seeing details clearly. Visual acuity scores are expressed as a fraction, not a percentage.

Normal vision is 6/6 (in metres) or 20/20 (in feet). The first number of the fraction represents the patient's distance from the Snellen chart. The second number shows the distance from which most people without a visual impairment would be able to read the line of letters on the chart (see box, *Visual impairment*).

Eye examination

An eye examination will show if there are other causes of diminished vision, such as age-related macular degeneration (AMD), cataracts, glaucoma or other eye diseases. It includes an external examination of the eye and its adnexa (eyelids, tear glands and tear ducts), an evaluation of ocular motility (an eye that deviates, excessive movement, etc.), a biomicroscopic examination (for detecting cataracts, vitreous hemorrhage, etc.) and intraocular pressure measurement.

Fundus examination

A diagnosis of DR is made by an optometrist or an ophthalmologist based on an examination of the back of the eye (the fundus), which makes it possible to evaluate the condition of the retina. There are different ways of performing this examination: it can be done with an ophthalmoscope or a biomicroscope (slit-lamp), with or without contact lenses. The patient's pupil must be dilated.

A fundus examination is not painful. It allows the vision specialist to see characteristic signs of DR, such as presence of microaneurysms, macular edema or more serious lesions in the retina (hemorrhages or neovascularization). With this information, the type of DR (proliferative or nonproliferative) can generally be deter mined and a decision can be made about what to do next (*Figure* ❶

FUNDUS PHOTOGRAPHY

Though still not routinely used in all doctors' offices, fundus photogra phy is an innovative tool with much promise for the future of telemed icine (remote diagnosis and treatment by means of telecommunication and information technology). Digital colour photos are taken of the back of the eye (retinal photos taken with a fundus camera). Fundus photography is becoming the preferred screening method because allows an ophthalmologist to evaluate a patient remotely (telediagno sis). Photographs of the eye can be taken by a technician and ther sent to an ophthalmologist for diagnosis—a tremendous help in fo lowing patients living in remote areas. In addition, doctors can keep the photos and compare them with photos taken at a later date to track the progression of the disease. Fundus photography is painless In addition, unlike fundus examination with an ophthalmoscope or slit lamp, fundus photography allows examination of the retina with out systematic pupil dilation.

PUPIL DILATION

Pupil dilation is required for a proper fundus examination as well as for fluorescein angiography. Drops are put in the eye to force the pupil to stay open. It takes about 15 minutes for the drops to take full effect. Pupil dilation is not painful, but the eyes may become sensitive to light and near vision can be disturbed for several hours. It is thus recommended that the patient bring a pair of sunglasses and either be accompanied or make arrangements for the trip home. Patients are advised not to drive for several hours after the examination.

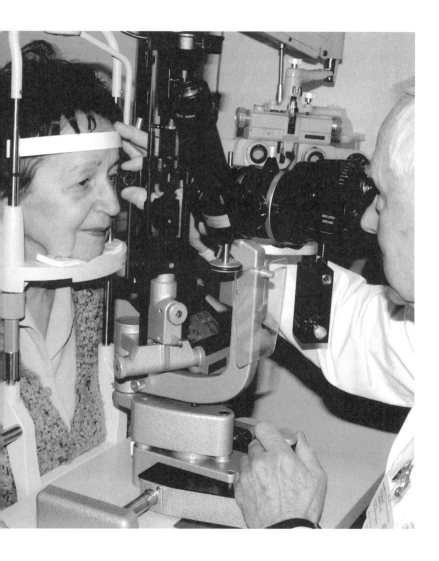

Slit-lamp examination

OPTICAL COHERENCE TOMOGRAPHY (OCT)

Optical coherence tomography, or OCT, is like an ultrasound, except light is used instead of sound. The OCT scanner measures the time it takes for the light (its speed) to travel through the ocular media and the retina before it is reflected back by tissues and structures. These measurements are used to generate cross-sectional images of the back of the eye (the ocular fundus), from the outermost to the deepest layers.

OCT is used to measure the thickness of the retina and hence indicates presence or absence of retinal edema, which is characteristic of DR. Within minutes, the ophthalmologist can also detect any macular edema, painlessly and without injection.

OCT is currently used to diagnose and follow patients with DR. It is very helpful in evaluating treatment efficacy, as it allows measurement of retina thickness. If necessary, physicians will use fluorescein angiography, which provides information that complements that obtained with OCT (*Figure* ❷).

FLUORESCEIN ANGIOGRAPHY

Fluorescein angiography is a technique for examining blood circulation in the retina by injecting a dye (fluorescein or indocyanine green) into a vein. It is used to check for complications of DR (edema, hemorrhages, etc.). However, it is mainly used to determine if a patient has proliferative or nonproliferative DR, as it can confirm the presence and extent of neovascularization and the location of the new abnormal blood vessels (*Figure* ❸). Fluorescein angiography and OCT are more accurate than a fundus examination. However, fluorescein angiography is becoming less and less popular with ophthalmologists, who prefer OCT because it does not require injection of dye. Fluorescein angiography is mainly used to complement OCT when required.

For this test, like the fundus examination, the pupil is dilated with eye drops. The dye injected into a vein in the patient's forearm or

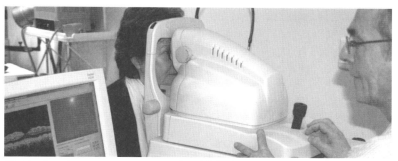

Optical coherence tomography (OCT) scanner

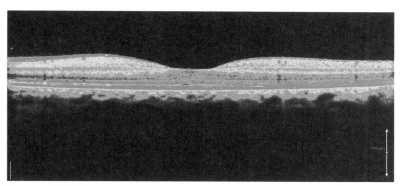

Normal OCT scan

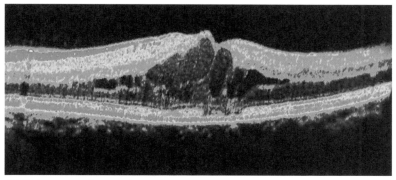

OCT image of macular edema

❷

hand quickly reaches the eye and colours the vessels at the back of the eye. The ophthalmic photographer or technician then takes a series of photos using a camera equipped with special filters.

Fluorescein is the dye most frequently used, and the examination takes only a few minutes. It is rarely necessary to use indocyanine green, which allows examination of deeper layers (choroid).

Adverse effects of dyes

Adverse effects of angiography are rare and generally not harmful. Fluorescein can provoke nausea, dizziness and sometimes vomiting. When these effects occur, they do so within minutes of the injection of the dye and disappear just as rapidly.

Strong allergic reactions to fluorescein (anaphylaxis) are extremely rare.

Fluorescein in the blood stream colours the skin and the whites of the eyes an orangey yellow. This discoloration appears a few minutes after the dye is injected and lasts for several hours. The urine will also appear dark yellow or orange for about 24 hours.

Indocyanine green is well tolerated and does not cause nausea or vomiting. However, as it contains iodine, it must not be given to anyone with an iodine allergy. In addition, it is not recommended in the first three months of pregnancy.

Indocyanine green causes stools to turn green.

VISUAL IMPAIRMENT

Anyone whose visual acuity with an adequate optical correction is less than 6/21 (or 20/70) has a major visual impairment. This means the person can see at six metres (or 20 feet) an object that is generally perceived at 21 metres (or 70 feet) by someone with perfect vision.

If central vision is 6/60 (20/200) or less, the person is considered "legally blind."

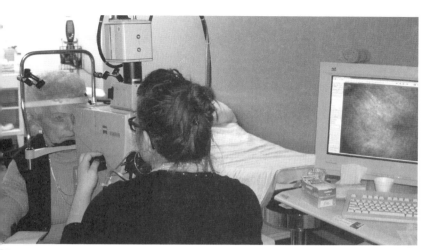

Fluorescein angiography equipment

Retinal blood
vessels

Macula

Optic nerve

Microaneurysms

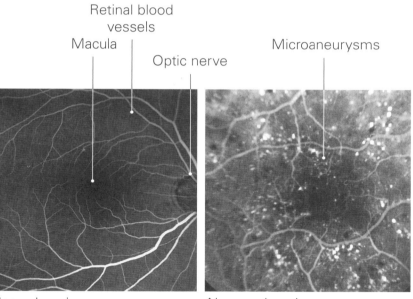

Normal angiogram

Abnormal angiogram

ULTRASOUND

Eye ultrasounds are rarely necessary in DR. They are only useful when media opacity (hemorrhage or cataract) makes it impossible to properly evaluate the ocular fundus with the other examinations, as ultrasound waves are not blocked by this opacity.

WHO DOES WHAT?

- An optician makes and sells corrective lenses based on a prescription written by an optometrist or an ophthalmologist. Opticians do not perform eye examinations.
- Optometrists are vision professionals but are not physicians. They are often the first practitioner consulted when vision problems arise. Based on a clinical eye examination, an optometrist can identify certain eye and vision problems, prescribe and/or sell glasses and, if need be, refer the patient to an ophthalmologist. In Quebec, an optometrist must refer the patient to a doctor (ophthalmologist or other physician) if he or she detects a problem that is not one of mild morbidity (that is, if he or she sees signs of disease).
- An ophthalmologist is a medical doctor. He or she is trained to perform a complete assessment of visual function, make diagnoses and provide medical and surgical treatment of diseases or disorders of the eye and related structures (eyelids, tear glands, tear ducts and eyeball).

ONE PERSON'S STORY

Name: Jonathan	**Age:** 18 years old

Occupation: Student

Jonathan has type 1 diabetes and has been treated with insulin since the age of 10. He controlled his disease very well for many years, but things changed in adolescence. He started to feel different from his friends and disease denial gradually took hold. Wanting to lead "a normal life," he began neglecting his therapy and refused to follow the recommended diet.

Shortly after turning 18, he noticed that he was having difficulty seeing objects that were far away. He figured he needed glasses, so he consulted an optometrist—who determined he was slightly myopic but also discovered retinal changes. The optometrist referred Jonathan to an ophthalmologist, who examined the back of Jonathan's eyes and diagnosed nonproliferative diabetic retinopathy (DR). To make sure there were no abnormal blood vessels (neovessels) on the retina, the ophthalmologist used fluorescein angiography. This test confirmed that there were no neovessels on the retina, and optical coherence tomography (OCT) showed there was no macular edema. The ophthalmologist thus concluded that Jonathan's myopia was caused by elevated blood sugar (hyperglycemia). As this condition is reversible, the ophthalmologist advised Jonathan to see his family doctor to gain better control of his diabetes.

Jonathan has gradually regained his normal vision and has considerably reduced the risk of his diabetic retinopathy progressing to the proliferative stage thanks to better management of his diabetes. He has also understood that diabetes is not incompatible with a happy life.

CHAPTER 5
PREVENTION
AND TREATMENT

Though prevention, through regular eye examinations and satisfactory diabetes management, is the best way to avoid or slow the progression of diabetic retinopathy (DR), different therapeutic options are available depending on the stage of the disease. For nonproliferative DR without macular edema, no treatment is required. For proliferative DR and complications of DR, particularly macular edema, there are a number of treatments and the ophthalmologist will decide which is most appropriate for the situation. New treatments available in the last few years have greatly improved outcomes.

PREVENTING OR SLOWING THE PROGRESSION OF DR

When a diagnosis of diabetes is received, the patient will want to do everything possible to prevent diabetic retinopathy, slow its progression and maintain good vision. The best way is to target the main risk factors for diabetes—elevated blood sugar, but also high blood pressure and elevated cholesterol. It is also important to remember that DR can be asymptomatic until it reaches a very advanced stage. Disease prevention measures and regular monitoring of the back of the eye are thus crucial elements that must not be neglected by anyone with type 1 or type 2 diabetes.

Control your blood sugar

Optimal blood sugar control remains the best way to prevent the onset of DR and slow its progression. It has been clearly demonstrated that DR incidence increases with blood sugar imbalance, in type 1 as well as type 2 diabetes. Maintaining a blood sugar level as close to normal as possible is thus essential. To achieve this, some diabetics must take medication (oral hypoglycemic drugs or insulin injections). The attending physician will decide what is appropriate.

Control your blood pressure

Controlling blood pressure can slow the progression of DR and thus reduce the risk of vision loss in people who are diabetic and have high blood pressure. Furthermore, the changes to the retina that high blood pressure causes (hypertensive retinopathy) can make it more difficult and riskier to treat DR.

In addition to drug therapy, regular exercise, smoking cessation and an appropriate diet can help to stabilize blood pressure.

Control your cholesterol

As hypercholesterolemia is a known risk factor for DR (*see Chapter 3*), good control of blood cholesterol level is crucial in diabetics to prevent onset or aggravation of DR. Recommendations for reducing blood cholesterol are to cut back on red meat, choose low-fat dairy products, use olive oil instead of butter or margarine, limit coffee consumption, eat more fibre, exercise and lose all excess weight. Drug therapy is often necessary as well.

Eat a balanced diet

Diabetics require a balanced diet. Sugars must be avoided, as they will cause a rapid rise in blood sugar level. With an appropriate diet, people with diabetes reduce the risk of developing complications of diabetes such as DR.

Maintain a healthy weight

In people with diabetes, excess weight increases the risk of developing DR. It is important to exercise regularly and follow the recommendations of *Canada's Food Guide*. These measures are also good for the heart. It can also be worthwhile to consult a nutritionist.

Have regular eye examinations

The Canadian Ophthalmological Society recommends regular eye examinations by an ophthalmologist or an optometrist, the frequency depending on the severity of the DR: every year in case of early nonproliferative DR but more frequently (every three to six months) in case of advanced DR. The ophthalmologist or optometrist will determine how long to wait between eye exams.

Quit smoking

It has been demonstrated that diabetics who smoke are more susceptible than diabetics who do not smoke to diabetes complications, particularly the onset of DR or the progression of existing DR. These complications arise because tobacco damages the blood vessels. Smoking cessation thus helps to prevent the progression of DR. There are a number of effective ways to quit smoking. A doctor or a pharmacist can provide additional information.

TREATING DR

No treatment is indicated, at present, for nonproliferative DR without macular edema. Prevention is still the best way to maintain good vision. Of course, regular eye examinations are also important, for early identification of complications or progression to a more advanced stage.

In case of proliferative DR, or complications such as macular edema, vitreous hemorrhage, neovascular glaucoma or retinal detachment, different treatments are possible, alone or in combination: laser photocoagulation, antiangiogenic drugs, corticosteroids or vitrectomy. The ophthalmologist will decide which treatment is appropriate depending on the patient's condition.

Laser photocoagulation

Laser photocoagulation can be local (focal photocoagulation) or more extensive (scatter or panretinal photocoagulation, PRP).

Laser light of a very specific wavelength is absorbed by the retina and converted into heat. This heat destroys (burns) certain cells, including those that produce vascular endothelial growth factor (VEGF), which is responsible for neovascularization. The result? Regression of neovascularization, reducing the risk of complications such as vitreous hemorrhage.

Laser photocoagulation is indicated in most cases of proliferative DR and sometimes for treatment of certain cases of macular edema. It is also used during vitrectomy (discussed later in this chapter). In addition, it can be used to treat neovascular glaucoma, one of the more serious complications of DR, in combination with other therapies such as antiangiogenic injections, filtration surgery, ciliary body photocoagulation, cryotherapy and endocyclophotocoagulation.

The ophthalmologist will decide when treatment should be introduced based on signs observed. The number of sessions required to complete the treatment depends on the severity of the diabetic retinopathy. If there is a very large number of abnormal blood vessels, then more laser shots will be required.

In case of macular edema or vitreous hemorrhage, the doctor may decide to administer antiangiogenic injections (*see Antiangiogenics, below*) before undertaking laser photocoagulation therapy. Laser therapy cannot be used if there is too much blood in the vitreous. Antiangiogenic injections will stop further bleeding so that laser photocoagulation therapy can be started when the blood is sufficiently resorbed.

Laser photocoagulation will generally put a stop to neovascularization for an undetermined period. The number of sessions required to achieve this result differs from one patient to the next, but the stability achieved can last for years, sometimes decades.

Laser photocoagulation can considerably reduce the risk of blindness associated with DR by stabilizing vision. In some cases of localized macular edema, it can even improve vision.

How is the treatment given?

Laser photocoagulation is performed under local anesthesia in a hospital or in the ophthalmologist's office. Only the surface of the eye is anesthetized, with eye drops. In very rare cases, the doctor will deem it necessary to anesthetize the entire eye with an injection.

In preparation for the procedure, eye drops are placed in the eye to dilate the pupil. The doctor then makes a number of laser shots (microscopic burns) to the area of the retina that requires treatment. The number of laser shots varies depending on whether the treatment is focal or panretinal (*see above*). In some cases, hundreds may be made in a session.

The procedure lasts from five to 30 minutes. The patient may experience glare, mainly at the start of the treatment, and sometimes mild pain. Most people say they experienced some discomfort.

Two or three sessions per eye are sometimes required. Several weeks are allowed to elapse between sessions, and the ophthalmologist generally treats only one eye in any one session. The therapy ends when examination of the back of the eye shows that the neovascularization has disappeared, at which point the DR is considered inactive. Follow-up is none-theless required.

The patient can return home right after the treatment and resume his or her usual activities. However, the patient should be accompanied on leaving the ophthalmology clinic. He or she should not drive after the treatment because of the pupil dilation and should refrain from physical effort.

Eye drops are sometimes prescribed to reduce the inflammation caused by the treatment.

Side effects

The main adverse effect is edema of the retina, sometimes including the macula. Even though laser photocoagulation can be used to treat macular edema, it can actually cause it if the treatment is too aggressive. This is why the doctor spreads the treatment over several sessions, to minimize the swelling.

Mild headache may also be experienced in the hours following the treatment. As the treatment can cause stress in diabetics, blood sugar level may rise temporarily. However, there is no cause for concern, as it will return to normal rapidly.

On the other hand, the greater the number of laser shots made, the bigger the risk that the treatment will cause a loss of side vision (peripheral vision) and slower dark adaptation. These side effects are often temporary, with normal vision restored in the weeks or even days following the treatment. These are not complications, just predictable effects that the ophthalmologist can discuss with the patient before undertaking the treatment. These side effects can become permanent in rare cases when the disease is extremely advanced and abnormal blood vessels cover a very large area of the retina and have even invaded the vitreous. At this advanced stage of the disease, treatment has to be more aggressive and may cause permanent peripheral vision loss (central vision will be preserved, as the treatment does not target the macula) and permanent decrease in dark adaptation. Laser treatment sometimes affects night vision, as it can damage the rods, the extremely light-sensitive photoreceptors in the retina (*see Chapter 1*). The patient might have difficulty finding a seat in a dark movie theatre, for example.

Antiangiogenics

Researchers made a major breakthrough in late 2004 with the use of antiangiogenics, or antivascular endothelial growth factor (anti-VEGF) agents, in the treatment of a number of eye diseases, including diabetic retinopathy. These drugs neutralize the activity of vascular endothelial growth factor or VEGF, which triggers the growth of new abnormal blood vessels and the associated swelling. Injected directly into the eye, these agents can stabilize DR and slow its progression.

Antiangiogenic injections are used mainly to treat macular edema in nonproliferative or proliferative DR. They are sometimes used in combination with other therapies to obtain better results. In case of vitreous hemorrhage or neovascular glaucoma (two complications of proliferative DR), antiangiogenic injections can be used to stop the hemorrhaging before undertaking laser photocoagulation therapy (*see Laser photocoagulation, above*). The ophthalmologist may also decide to administer antiangiogenic injections before a vitrectomy (*see Vitrectomy, below*), to prevent recurrence of hemorrhages after the operation.

Two antiangiogenic agents are currently available in Canada to treat DR, ranibizumab (Lucentis®) and bevacizumab (Avastin®), but only ranibizumab is recognized by Health Canada for ophthalmological use.

In case of macular edema, antiangiogenic injections will generally improve or at least stabilize vision. However, ophthalmological monitoring is required at a frequency prescribed by the doctor, as macular edema can reappear.

How is the treatment given?

The treatment is given in the doctor's office or a hospital. The patient must not wear makeup on the day of the treatment, to reduce the risk of infection. Before the injection, the patient generally undergoes an imaging test (OCT) (*see Chapter 4*) to give the doctor an accurate picture of the condition of the retina. The eye is then disinfected with antiseptic solution and locally anesthetized using eye drops or a small subconjunctival injection. An eyelid speculum is used to keep the eye open as the antiangiogenic agent is injected into the white of the eye. This only takes a few seconds. The procedure is not painful and is well tolerated by patients.

The therapy generally consists in a series of monthly injections (usually three or four in all). The number of injections depends on the progression of the macular edema, which the ophthalmologist determines based on the OCT exam.

The ophthalmologist will sometimes recommend that antibiotic drops be used for several days after the injection to prevent infection. The ophthalmologist will also prescribe artificial tears, eye drops to be used for a limited time in the treated eye to relieve irritation caused by the disinfectant. The patient can resume his or her usual activities on the same day, or the following day.

Side effects

Complications stemming from injections to the eye are very rare. It is normal for the eye to be mildly irritated following the treatment. A temporary elevation of intraocular pressure is also possible but is generally without consequences. In very rare cases, an infection can occur inside the eyeball (endophthalmitis), in which case the eye becomes red and very painful, there is significant vision loss, and an emergency trip to the hospital is required.

Corticosteroids

A common treatment for macular edema only a few years ago, corticosteroids are a less and less popular treatment option since the arrival of anti-VEGF, demonstrated to be effective in numerous clinical studies. Though corticosteroids have been shown to be effective, they are a less attractive option as side effects are frequent and substantial. Corticosteroids are still useful, however, when anti-VEGFs are contraindicated or have proved ineffective.

How is the treatment given?

The treatment is given in the same way as antiangiogenic injections (*see Antiangiogenics, above*).

Side effects

Common side effects of the treatment are eye irritation and temporary elevation of ocular pressure.

Cortisone can also cause clouding or opacification of the crystalline lens of the eye (cataracts). This is a relatively common side effect and requires surgery to remove the lens and replace it with an implant.

Cortisone can also cause changes to the eye that interfere with proper drainage of the aqueous humour, resulting in increased intraocular pressure (hypertonia) that can be permanent. This common side effect can be treated in different ways (drops, laser therapy or surgery) depending on the severity.

A more rare side effect is infection inside the eyeball (endophthalmitis), in which case the eye becomes red and very painful, there is significant vision loss and an emergency trip to the hospital is required.

Vitrectomy

Vitrectomy is a surgical procedure used mainly to treat two complications of proliferative DR: vitreous hemorrhage and retinal detachment.

Performed under local or general anesthesia, a vitrectomy consists in removing the vitreous humour of the eye (the transparent gel that fills the space between the crystalline lens and the retina). The vitreous humour is not essential for vision and can thus be removed and replaced by a transparent liquid or, temporarily, by gas.

When vitreous hemorrhaging persists after laser photocoagulation therapy, a vitrectomy can be performed to eliminate blood in the middle of the eye—the blood is removed at the same time as the vitreous gel, with which it is mixed.

In case of retinal detachment, vitrectomy removes the vitreou humour that is pulling on the retina. Once the vitreous humour i removed, different techniques are used to reattach the retina.

How is the treatment given?

The surgery is performed in a hospital, generally under loca anesthetic administered by injection close to the eye.

The ophthalmologist often administers laser photocoagula tion therapy during the vitrectomy to neutralize the abnorma blood vessels responsible for the vitreous hemorrhaging.

The patient can return home shortly after the vitrectomy, c after a night in hospital. Immobilization for several hours t several days is required.

The ophthalmologist will prescribe medicinal eye drops t protect the operated eye against infection. Wearing of eye prc tection (eye patch or shield) for a certain period is als recommended.

Vision recovery after vitrectomy is variable and can tak several weeks.

Side effects

A common complication of vitrectomy is redness and sensitiv ity of the eye for several days after the surgery. The crystalline lens may become cloudy or opacified (cataract), especiall when gas is used. This can be treated with surgery, dependin on the extent of the opacification.

Of course, there are risks with any surgery. In rare cases vitrectomy can lead to infection, retinal detachment, macula edema or, in extreme cases, loss of vision in the operated eye

Emergency consultation of an ophthalmologist is recom mended after vitrectomy in case of vision loss, eye pain or pei sistent redness of the eye.

ONE PERSON'S STORY

Name: Geraldine

Age: 76 years old

Occupation: Retired

Ten years ago, at the age of 66, Geraldine learned she had type 2 diabetes. She must have had it for some time without being aware of it, as she already had nonproliferative DR at the time of the diagnosis. Six years later, Geraldine underwent laser photocoagulation therapy in both eyes, as the DR had become proliferative. However, even at this advanced stage of the disease, she didn't perceive any vision loss and was able to continue her normal activities.

Over the last year, however, she noticed a gradual loss of vision. She was finding it more and more difficult to read and watch television. Though she wasn't concerned at first, attributing the vision loss to fatigue, she decided to consult a doctor when she realized her vision was not returning to normal. On examining Geraldine's eyes, the ophthalmologist discovered that her vision was 6/30 (20/100) in the right eye and so diminished in the left eye that she was unable to count fingers held in front of the eye at a distance of more than 50 centimetres. Examination of the back of the eye showed severe macular edema in the right eye, confirmed by optical coherence tomography (OCT). The retina of the left eye, however, could not be examined because the vitreous was filled with blood.

Geraldine and her doctor discussed the results of the examination and decided to treat the macular edema of the right eye with anti-angiogenic (ranibizumab) injections at four-week intervals. Geraldine's vision in this eye improved significantly after several treatments (to 6/15 or 20/50), while the left eye started to clear up by itself, without treatment. A decision was thus made to wait a while before treating the left eye, but a vitrectomy will most likely be required to remove blood from the vitreous.

CHAPTER 6
LIVING WITH
DIABETIC
RETINOPATHY

A diagnosis of diabetic retinopathy (DR) does not mean you will eventually go blind. It does, however, require adaptation to a new situation, especially when the DR is accompanied by vision loss. Whether sudden or gradual, vision loss entails functional, physical and even sometimes psychological challenges for those who experience it. Fortunately, there are many optical, electronic and computerized aids as well as vision, orientation and mobility rehabilitation programs to help those affected remain independent.

Vision rehabilitation centres offer a range of services, including assessment of functional vision and help in maintaining and optimizing independent reading, writing and getting around. In many cases, these services even make it possible for people with DR to take courses, keep their jobs or find an accommodated job. After the initial shock of learning one's vision is impaired and a transition period that can be long or short, the vast majority of people with DR are able to adjust to their new condition.

LOW VISION REHABILITATION

When there is a major loss of vision, the patient with DR can enter a vision rehabilitation program in a specialized centre to learn how to use his or her remaining vision. The program will vary depending on the type of vision loss. Some people with DR have reduced visual acuity, while others lose vision in the peripheral and/or central visual field. These different types of visual loss are often concomitant, that is, they appear simultaneously.

In Canada, vision rehabilitation services are offered free of charge based on certain criteria (field of vision affected, visual acuity, etc.).

Eccentric viewing training

This program teaches how to use eccentric vision (vision outside the macula). This is essential for rehabilitating people with DR when the macula, responsible for central vision, is affected. Eccentric viewing training helps people with DR learn to carry out the activities of daily living and to read and write. Instead of looking straight ahead, the person learns, through different exercises and tests, to use eccentric or peripheral vision. The preferred eccentric fixation point can be to the left or right, up or down, depending on the macular lesions. Different exercises are used to determine which area of eccentric vision gives the clearest image.

The rehabilitation generally takes several months. However, it is impossible to say with any accuracy exactly how long it will take as it depends on the damage to the macula, the visual needs of the person and the speed of assimilation of the techniques taught. The training can sometimes cause fatigue or headaches, but it is important not to get discouraged.

By the end of the rehabilitation period, the person with DR will have optimized his or her remaining vision.

VISION AIDS AND OTHER USEFUL PRODUCTS

Having a vision impairment or "low vision" does not mean you are blind. Almost everyone with DR has some remaining vision that can be optimized with the help of vision aids. Optometrists or ophthalmologists can recommend and prescribe vision aids based on the residual vision, capabilities and visual needs of the person with DR. Some vision aids are used only for near vision, others are for far vision and still others are multifunctional.

Some provinces have financial assistance programs for procurement of these assistive devices. Eligibility criteria include visual acuity and/or field of vision impairment, income, benefit and retirement plans, age and occupational status. Vision aids can be loaned to eligible people or purchased from stores that specialize in adaptive products.

All of these vision aids require an adjustment and learning period, as they alter the vision habits of those who use them. Vision rehabilitation centres support users through this learning process, and vision rehabilitation specialists teach them strategies for optimal use of prescribed vision aids.

Vision aids

Different optical systems use special lenses to enlarge the image for reading or writing.

Magnifiers

Magnifiers come in different shapes, strengths and sizes. Some have a built-in adjustable lighting system (incandescent, halogen or LED). There are handheld and pocket magnifiers, bar magnifiers and stand magnifiers (*Figure* ❶).

Closed-circuit televisions (CCTVs)

These devices use video technology to magnify letters to the desired size for reading and project them onto a screen. Contrast and brightness can be adjusted. CCTVs have a tray on which the book, magazine or document to be read is placed and a screen above it where the text is displayed in the character size selected by the user. CCTVs can also be used for writing or performing manual tasks requiring fine detail vision (*Figure* ❷).

Electronic glasses

These lightweight, battery-operated glasses provide up to 30 times magnification. They are used for theatre, cinema or television and can be converted to a standard magnifier for reading or writing. They transmit magnified, real-time, colour images of both near and far objects.

Telescopes

A small telescope can be clipped onto one or both lenses of a pair of glasses as needed to make objects that are far away or in the intermediate distance appear larger. These devices are very useful when travelling—for reading signs in the subway, for example. Binocular telescopic systems (for both eyes) are used like a pair of binoculars to see things at a distance or to watch television. Telescopes mounted on glasses can be used to take courses or watch shows (*Figure* ❸).

Computer applications

Different software makes it possible to read or write documents on a computer.

Screen readers

These programs convert printed documents (books, newspaper articles, etc.) that have been scanned into electronic documents that can be saved on a computer. The programs can even read electronic documents out loud, magnify the text on screen and modify the colour contrast to improve visibility.

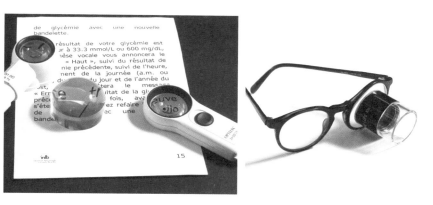

❶ Magnifiers and other near vision aids

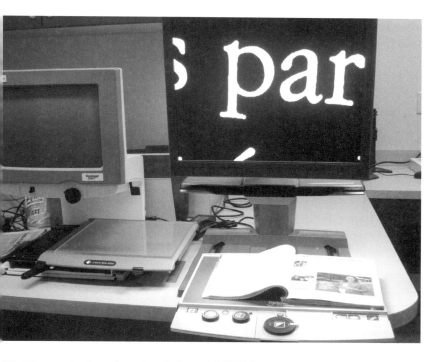

❷ Closed-circuit television (CCTV)

Screen magnifiers

These programs magnify text, graphics and images displayed on a computer screen. Some screen magnifiers also magnify the mouse pointer and text cursor, and others allow the user to adjust the degree of magnification. Screen magnifiers are especially helpful for surfing the Internet (*Figure* ❹).

Assistive devices for daily living

A variety of assistive devices facilitate everyday life for people with visual impairments. These include clocks with large numbers, big-button telephones, TV remote controls and magnifying screens, knitting/crocheting aids, talking thermostats and adapted kitchenware (knives, high-contrast tableware (half black, half white), audible liquid level indicators, etc.).

Healthcare devices and accessories for people with diabetes

A number of devices are available to facilitate healthcare for people with diabetes who have a visual impairment, including insulin pens, syringes with large numbers, medication organizers, talking glucometers and talking scales.

ADAPTING THE HOME

Certain home adaptations can improve the comfort and safety of people with DR and help them stay in their own homes and remain independent. Sometimes it's just a question of adjusting the lighting to make the home functional, as people with DR need more lighting to enhance contrasts.

The vision rehabilitation specialist will rarely recommend that a person with DR move, unless access to the home is unsafe (too many steps, for example) and the person's mobility is reduced. Instead, the ergonomics of the living space of the person with DR is organized based on his or her remaining vision, visual acuity and visual field impairment. The adaptation may consist in putting

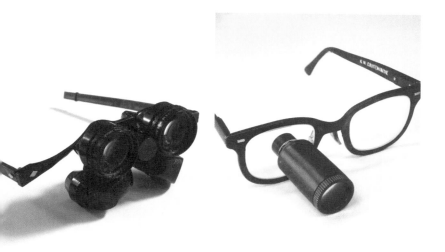

❸ Binocular and monocular telescopic systems

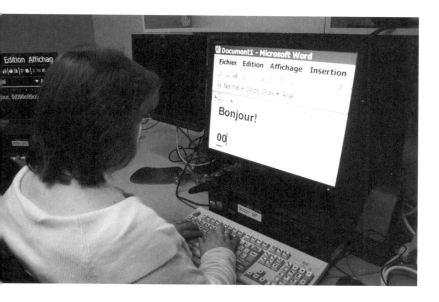

❹ Screen magnifier

reflective strips on stair treads to mark the beginning and end of each step, making locks more accessible or using orange tactile stickers to mark the most commonly used temperatures on the stove. Bathrooms can also be adapted to make then safer for personal care and daily hygiene.

ADAPTING THE WORKPLACE

Employers are more and more open to the idea of adapting the workplace, when possible, to keep employees with DR who have suffered vision loss as a result of complications. In Quebec, if you are eligible for the government assistance program, a vision rehabilitation specialist will even meet with your employer to help assess your work station. Software to magnify text and images on a computer screen and speech generating devices can also be borrowed. If you are unable to keep your job, you will be offered career counselling services and training programs to help you find a new job better suited to your condition.

GETTING AROUND

Anyone living with a visual impairment has special needs and varying degrees of difficulty getting around. When the impairment is due to DR, travelling is often more difficult because of the visual field loss, the reduced visual acuity and the contrast loss. In addition, there is more difficulty adapting to changes in brightness when moving from an indoor to an outdoor space or vice versa. Lighting conditions of different environments have a huge effect on the vision of a person with DR, as they require adaptation. Nonetheless, it is important to remember that even with low vision travel is possible—alone or with assistance, on foot or by taxi, public transit or paratransit. To be able to travel independently, all that is required is to use existing resources and the services of the orientation and mobility specialists at the vision rehabilitation centres.

On foot

When visual impairment makes getting around on foot less safe or more difficult, a white cane (for support or identification) or accompaniment is a solution. A white cane is not required with DR, but some people feel more secure with a cane and use it to locate steps and obstacles. Others like to carry a white cane to alert strangers to their visual impairment.

Assistance from a friend or family member can be helpful when travelling to unknown places or in crowded areas. People with DR whose peripheral visual field is reduced will want a cane when travelling.

Public transit

Many people with DR use public transit daily. Subways are often more difficult than buses for people with severe visual impairments. The lighting is not the same from one station to the next, and accesses are totally different—with corridors and stairways of varying lengths. If the same route is taken regularly, it can be learned, so it becomes a familiar routine with known obstacles. An orientation and mobility specialist can help with this travel training. He or she will make the trip with you and help you work out the easiest and safest strategies for that particular route.

Anyone with a visual acuity of 6/60 (20/200) or less, or a field of vision of 20 degrees or less, can obtain a blind ID card from the Canadian National Institute for the Blind (CNIB). This ID card entitles the holder to discounts on many public transit services.

Some non-profit organizations also provide transportation services with volunteer chauffeurs who drive their own cars. Last but not least, taxis or paratransit are good options when other ways of getting around seem complicated or unsafe.

By car

A diagnosis of DR does not necessarily mean losing your driver's licence. Conditions for retaining a driver's licence vary in Canada from one province to the next. In Quebec, visual acuity must be at least 6/15 (20/50) with both eyes open and examined together to be able to drive a road vehicle.

Sometimes the ophthalmologist or optometrist will ask a patient to hand over his or her driver's licence. However, if the patient's vision improves enough with treatment, the licence may be returned. In this respect, good diabetes management without episodes of severe hypoglycemia is important in the months preceding the request to have a driver's licence renewed.

At any rate, it is best to avoid driving at night, when there isn't much contrast and the risk of blinding by headlights is higher.

DON'T BE BLINDED BY LIGHT

Some people with DR are easily blinded by sunlight or glare. Goggles, which offer lateral protection, are thus recommended. Some models have contrast enhancement filters. Recently, manufacturers have been making an effort to improve the look of these goggles, and more and more models are available.

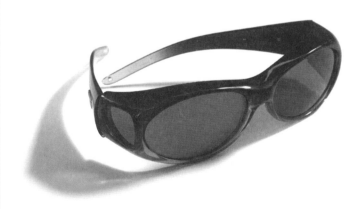

Goggles

As an alternative, paratransit services are offered in most parts of Canada.

HELP FROM FAMILY AND FRIENDS

DR can have a major psychological impact. It affects not only your mobility and independence but also your self-image. In some cases, when DR is diagnosed at the same time as diabetes, the patient must adapt to a new lifestyle requiring a restrictive diet and specialized care in addition to getting used to a possible vision loss. Support from close friends and family members is crucial. Friends and family, who are often very upset by the diagnosis, can receive advice and explanations during a visit to the optometrist or ophthalmologist, or a meeting with a vision rehabilitation specialist.

The friends and family of a person with DR are the first to want to help with daily living activities and to be available to do so. However, they may tend to do things for you, especially if they don't know what you can do by yourself. It's best if they offer help, which you can refuse if you don't need it, instead of just doing things for you.

The reactions of friends and family are crucial for the person with DR. They can affect your self-esteem and rehabilitation. If you feel that your family does not accept your condition, you will have difficulty accepting it yourself and making the necessary effort to remain independent. Worse yet, certain reactions can affect your feelings of self-worth and lead to depression. This is why it is so important that family and friends support and encourage the person with DR.

SPECIALIZED PSYCHOSOCIAL SERVICES

The emotional aspect of vision loss is one of the biggest difficulties to overcome. When you learn you have DR, you may experience many emotions—shock, denial, anger, rage, sadness, etc. These may occur in any order and with any intensity, and may last for any length of time. Some people relive the different stages of grief with every vision change, even when they are prepared and have been through it before.

A person with DR may even go through a period of depression, in which case help must be found. Support groups and organizations that provide psychological assistance are available for people with DR (*see Useful Addresses*). Your eye specialist will even refer you to a psychologist if you feel the need. However, the services offered in a vision rehabilitation centre, together with low vision monitoring, are often enough to dispel worries and fears and move past the initial state of shock. One thing is certain: accepting the disease helps the person with DR to adjust to the changes and remain confident and independent.

ONE PERSON'S STORY

Name: Jack	**Âge:** 57 years old

Occupation: Truck driver

Despite numerous warnings from his family doctor, Jack never took the diagnosis of type 2 diabetes he received in his forties seriously and did not follow his doctor's recommendations. He didn't want to change his lifestyle. He didn't want to stop eating foods that he liked, sweets in particular, just because he had been diagnosed with diabetes. Sometime after his 55th birthday, he noticed a gradual loss of vision and decided to consult an ophthalmologist. The ophthalmologist told him he had diabetic retinopathy and that it had reached a very advanced stage. With treatment, he was able to recover some of the vision he had lost, but his central vision remained impaired. He lost his driver's licence as a result of the vision impairment and was no longer able to work as a truck driver.

These sudden changes were very hard to accept. However, with the help of his wife and children, Jack stepped up to the plate and was eventually able to accept the situation. A vision rehabilitation specialist helped him adapt his home and an orientation and mobility specialist taught him travel skills so he could take the bus to work. Jack feels he has a very good chance of finding a job suited to his condition in the company where he worked as a truck driver. He has received training in eccentric viewing and is ready for a warehouse inventory management position where he would use a computer with adapted software.

Jack plans to take care of his health in the future so he can preserve his eccentric vision, which was spared by the disease. He has changed his lifestyle and is now following the recommendations his doctor made so many years ago.

CHAPTER 7

TREATMENTS
OF THE FUTURE

Given the high incidence of diabetic retinopathy (DR) among diabetics, DR research is very active at present and has substantial financial support. Advances are being made rapidly, giving hope that future treatments will be even more effective in limiting complications and repairing lesions. With the extraordinary progress in research on new therapies, no one can predict today how DR will be treated ten or even five years from now. In fact, new therapeutic options have recently become available for macular edema. For close to 35 years, laser therapy was the gold standard for this complication of DR, but recent clinical studies have demonstrated the superiority of antiangiogenic injections in most cases. Now more than ever, the future looks promising, not only for early diagnosis and rapid treatment of DR but also for the possibility of repairing eyes damaged by the disease.

FUTURE DRUGS

In the years ahead, new drugs now being studied may offer treatment for DR at an earlier stage. A number of pharmaceutical companies are working on the development these drugs, and several clinical trials have already been conducted. These new drugs will probably be able to prevent neovascularization and cause DR to regress, reducing the need for laser therapy and surgery.

FUTURE ANTIANGIOGENIC THERAPIES

Current research is directed mainly at improving existing treatments for macular edema and proliferative DR. Doctors now have medications that can be injected into the vitreous humour of the eye. These antiangiogenic (or anti-VEGF) therapies cause swellings to stabilize and even regress. However, the injections have to be repeated every month for a certain period of time. Researchers are keenly interested in developing sustained-release delivery systems so antiangiogenics can act continuously. One option being studied is implantation in the vitreous body of biodegradable capsules containing extended-release antiangiogenic agents.

New anti-VEGF drugs are expected on the market in the very near future. One such class of drugs, the VEGF-Trap, prevents VEGF from binding to its receptors and is currently undergoing licensing review in Canada. With these drugs, less frequent eye injections will be required. Other new drugs under study include SiRNAs, which are anti-VEGF medications that suppress VEGF production. Many other anti-VEGF therapies are also under development. The goal is to develop new and more effective ways to prevent either the production or the action of VEGF.

GENE THERAPY

Gene therapy alters the genetic material of cells involved in disease. The structure of the defective gene in the cell is modified to prevent onset of the disease or make cells more resistant to it. Current gene therapy research is targeting not only eye diseases such as DR but also diabetes, the cause of DR, and other DR risk factors such as high blood pressure and hypercholesterolemia.

A viral vector is used to introduce a suitable genetic code. The virus must have the ability to penetrate the cell and insert its DNA in host chromosomes. The patient's cells can then produce the proteins that fight or correct diabetes or DR.

The challenge is to prevent disease progression by targeting the molecules involved. Researchers are trying to prevent the progression of diabetes by targeting genes that regulate insulin and altering cells of the pancreas so they start to secrete insulin again.

Gene therapy is a future treatment for prevention of DR. Additional studies are required to develop clinical applications. Though still in the experimental stage, gene therapies may nonetheless become available for people with DR in coming years.

STEM CELL TRANSPLANTATION

Retinal transplants are not a feasible option at present for people with DR. However, scientists hope to one day be able to repair retinal damage caused by DR by producing retinal cells and transplanting them in the eye. Some researchers believe stem cell transplantation will restore vision in people with DR. Transplantation of stem cells genetically modified to produce genes that protect against progression of DR is another possibility.

These procedures involve long-term research. We do not expect to be transplanting stem cells in the near future, as there are still technical problems. Nonetheless there is reason for much hope.

USEFUL ADDRESSES

CANADA

Canadian Association of Optometrists (CAO)
234 Argyle Avenue
Ottawa, ON K2P 1B9
1-613-235-7924 or 1-888-263-4676
www.opto.ca

Professional association of optometrists in Canada. It is also the national federation of 10 provincial associations of optometrists.

Canadian Diabetes Association
1400-522 University Avenue
Toronto, ON M5G 2R5
1-800-BANTING (1-800-226-8464)
www.diabetes.ca

Provides information, services and advice about diabetes and its management.

Canadian Ophthalmological Society
610-1525 Carling Avenue
Ottawa, ON K1Z 8R9
1-613-729-6779
www.eyesite.ca

Canadian association of physicians and surgeons specializing in eye care.

CNIB
1929 Bayview Avenue
Toronto, ON M4G 3E8
1-800-563-2642
www.cnib.ca

Nationwide, community-based, registered charity committed to research, public education and vision health for all Canadians.

CNIB Library
1929 Bayview Avenue
Toronto, ON M4G 3E8
1-800-563-2642
www.cnib.ca/en/services/library

Offers access to thousands of titles in Braille and PrintBraille as well as audio books, newspapers and magazine, descriptive videos and document search services. Alternate-media books and other documents can be consulted online or delivered on loan postage-free.

VoicePrint
1-800-567-6755
www.voiceprintcanada.com

A 24-hour reading service operated by the National Broadcast Reading Service. VoicePrint broadcasts readings of full-text articles 24/7 from more than 600 Canadian newspapers and magazines.

QUEBEC

Association des établissements de réadaptation en déficience physique du Québec (AERDPQ)
1001, boulevard de Maisonneuve Ouest, bureau 430
Montréal (QC) H3A 3C8
1-514-282-4205
www.aerdpq.org

Association of centres in the province of Quebec for rehabilitation of physical disabilities offering specialized rehabilitation services, for people with vision impairments in particular. Here is a list of centres by region.

Centre de protection et de réadaptation de la Côte-Nord
835, boulevard Jolliet
Baie-Comeau (QC) G5C 1P5
1-418-589-9927 or 1-866-389-2038
www.cprcn.qc.ca

Centre de réadaptation de la Gaspésie
230, route du Parc
Sainte-Anne-des-Monts (QC) G4V 2C4
1-418-763-3325 or 1-855-763-3325
www.crgaspesie.qc.ca

Centre de réadaptation en déficience physique Chaudière-Appalaches
9500, boulevard du Centre-Hospitalier
Charny (QC) G6X 0A1
1-418-380-2064
TDD: 1-418-380-2089
www.crdpca.qc.ca

Centre de réadaptation en déficience physique Le Bouclier
1075, boulevard Firestone, bureau 1000
Joliette (QC) J6E 6X6
1-450-755-2741 or 1-800-363-2783
TDD: 1-450-759-8763 or 1-877-870-8763
www.bouclier.qc.ca

Centre de réadaptation en déficience physique Le Parcours
2230, rue de l'Hôpital – C.P. 1200
Jonquière (QC) G7X 7X2
1-418-695-7700
TDD: 1-418-695-7839
www.csssjonquiere.qc.ca

Centre de réadaptation Estrie
300, rue King Est, bureau 200
Sherbrooke (QC) J1G 1B1
1-819-346-8411
TTY: 1-819-821-0247
www.centredereadaptationestrie.org

Centre de réadaptation InterVal
1775, rue Nicolas-Perrot
Trois-Rivières (QC) G9A 1C5
1-819-378-4083
www.centreinterval.qc.ca

Centre de réadaptation La Maison
100, chemin Docteur-Lemay
Rouyn-Noranda (QC) J9X 5T2
1-819-762-6592
www.crlm.qc.ca

Centre de réadaptation MAB-Mackay
7000, rue Sherbrooke Ouest
Montréal (QC) H4B 1R3
1-514-488-5552
www.mabmackay.ca

Centre régional de réadaptation La RessourSe
135, boulevard Saint-Raymond
Gatineau (QC) J8Y 6X7
1-819-777-6269
TTY: 1-819-777-0701
www.crr-la-ressourse.qc.ca

Centre régional de réadaptation L'interAction
800, avenue du Sanatorium
Mont-Joli (QC) G5H 3L6
1-418-775-7261 or 1-855-605-3235
www.csssmitis.ca/interaction

Institut de réadaptation en déficience physique de Québec (IRDPQ)
525, boulevard Wilfrid-Hamel
Québec (QC) G1M 2S8
1-418-529-9141
TDD/TTY: 1-418-649-3733
www.irdpq.qc.ca

Institut Nazareth & Louis-Braille
1111, rue Saint-Charles Ouest – Tour Ouest, 2e étage
Longueuil (QC) J4K 5G4
1-450-463-1710 or 1-800-361-7063
www.inlb.qc.ca

Consult the Web site for service points in Montreal, Laval and Saint-Jean-sur-Richelieu.

Association des médecins ophtalmologistes du Québec (AMOQ)

2, Complexe Desjardins – C.P. 216, succursale Desjardins
Montréal (QC) H5B 1G8
1-514-350-5124
www.amoq.org

Quebec association of ophthalmologists. The Web site provides information on diabetic retinopathy.

Association des optométristes du Québec (AOQ)

1265, rue Berri, bureau 740
Montréal (QC) H2L 4X4
1-514-288-6272 or 1-888-SOS-OPTO (1-888-767-6786)
www.aoqnet.qc.ca

Quebec association of optometrists. The Web site provides information for the public.

Audiothèque

4765, 1re Avenue, bureau 210
Québec (QC) G1H 2T3
1-418-627-8882
Montreal region: 1-514-393-0103 or 1-877-393-0103
www.audiotheque.com

Information centre for people who cannot access written materials. Offers telephone access to readings of newspaper articles, magazines, circulars and other written material.

Centre de réadaptation, d'orientation et d'intégration au travail (AIM CROIT)

750, boulevard Marcel-Laurin, bureau 450
Saint-Laurent (QC) H4M 2M4
1-514-744-2944
www.aimcroitqc.org

Accommodated job search assistance for people with visual impairments and workplace adaptation assistance for employers.

Comité d'adaptation de la main-d'oeuvre (CAMO)
55, avenue du Mont-Royal Ouest
Bureau 300, 3e étage
Montréal (QC) H2T 2S6
1-514-522-3310 or 1-888-522-3310
www.camo.qc.ca

Provincial committee whose mission is to promote access to training and employment for people living with disabilities.

CNIB
3044, rue Delisle
Montréal (QC) H4C 1M9
1-514-934-4622 or 1-800-465-4622
Quebec region: 1-418-204-1124
www.inca.ca

Nationwide, community-based, registered charity committed to research, public education and vision health for all Canadians.

Diabetes Québec
8550, boulevard Pie-IX, bureau 300
Montréal (QC) H1Z 4G2
1-514-259-3422 or 1-800-361-3504
www.diabete.qc.ca

Offers educational programs for people with diabetes and their families to help them learn more about diabetes and the best ways to control it. Publishes information and offers help and support.

Institut de réadaptation en déficience physique de Québec (IRDPQ)
525, boulevard Wilfrid-Hamel
Québec (QC) G1M 2S8
1-418-529-9141
www.irdpq.qc.ca

Offers a rehabilitation program for people with visual impairments and access to optical aids to compensate for visual loss.

Institut Nazareth & Louis-Braille (INLB)

1111, rue Saint-Charles Ouest – Tour Ouest, 2e étage
Longueuil (QC) J4K 5G4
1-450-463-1710 or 1-800-361-7063

Consult the Web site for service points in Montreal, Laval and Saint-Jean-sur-Richelieu.
www.inlb.qc.ca

Specializes in low vision rehabilitation. Member of the Association des établissements de réadaptation en déficience physique du Québec (AERDPQ). Offers services for people with total or partial vision loss.

Service québécois du livre adapté (SQLA)

475, boulevard De Maisonneuve Est
Montréal (QC) H2L 5C4
1-514-873-4454 or 1-866-410-0844
www.banq.qc.ca/sqla/index.html

A French-language adapted book collection (Braille and audio books) available at the Grande Bibliothèque.

Vues & Voies (formerly La Magnétothèque)

1055, boulevard René-Lévesque Est, bureau 501
Montréal (QC) H2L 4S5
1-514-282-1999 or 1-800-361-0635
www.vuesetvoix.com

Close to 10,000 audio books: novels, philosophy, psychology, biographies, etc. Volunteers also read editorials and articles from Quebec newspapers.

UNITED STATES

American Diabetes Association
1701 North Beauregard Street
Alexandria, VA 22311
1-800-342-2383
www.diabetes.org

WEB SITES

www.audible.com (in English)
www.audible.fr (in French)
Over 75,000 audiobooks available for download for a fee.

www.retinacanada.com
The Retina Foundation of Canada is dedicated to promoting public awareness and early detection of retinal diseases. Web site
provides information about diabetic retinopathy.